NEW THINKING ON IMPROVING MATERNITY CARE

International Perspectives

NEW THINKING ON IMPROVING MATERNITY CARE

International Perspectives

Edited by
Sarah Church
Lucy Frith
Marie-Clare Balaam
Marie Berg
Valerie Smith
Christa van der Walt
Soo Downe
Edwin van Teijlingen

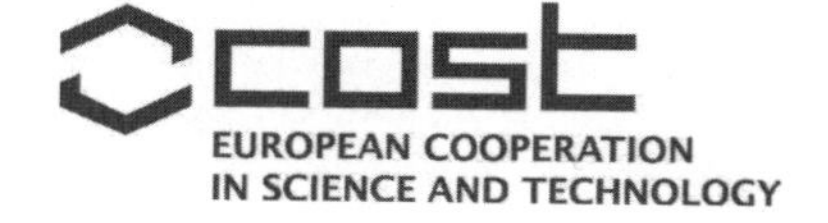

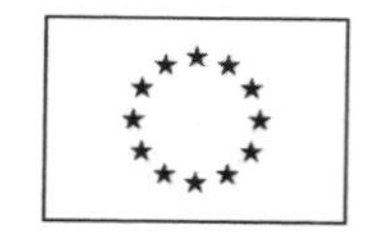

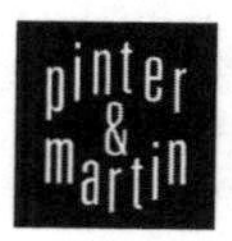

COST is supported by the EU Framework Programme Horizon 2020

COST (European Cooperation in Science and Technology) is a pan-European intergovernmental framework. Its mission is to enable breakthrough scientific and technological developments leading to new concepts and products and thereby contribute to strengthening Europe's research and innovation capacities. It allows researchers, engineers and scholars to jointly develop their own ideas and take new initiatives across all fields of science and technology, while promoting multi- and interdisciplinary approaches. COST aims at fostering a better integration of less research intensive countries to the knowledge hubs of the European Research Area. The COST Association, an international not-for-profit Association under Belgian law, integrates all management, governing and administrative functions necessary for the operation of the framework. The COST Association currently has 36 member countries. www.cost.eu

New Perspectives on International Maternity Care

First published by Pinter & Martin Ltd 2017

Cover image: *Mother and Child* by Virginia Day, photograph © Sinclair Jaspard Mandy, 2015.

ISBN 978-1-78066-240-4
Also available as ebook

British Library Cataloguing-in-Publication Data
A catalogue record for this book is available from the British Library.

Set in Palantino

Printed and bound in the UK by Ashford Colour Press Ltd, Godport, Hampshire

Pinter & Martin Ltd
6 Effra Parade
London SW2 1PS

pinterandmartin.com

Contents

FOREWORD

In 1997, Archie Cochrane awarded obstetrics a wooden spoon, for a lack of evidence-based practice. This critique was particularly focused on knowledge arising from randomised trials, but maternity care was equally unresponsive to the body of anthropological and sociological research that had been growing since the 1970s, particularly from feminist researchers of various persuasions. While the wooden spoon award spurred the development of the Cochrane Collaboration (starting with the Pregnancy and Childbirth database), and, ultimately, the evidence-based medicine (EBM) movement, there is still a gap between researchers investigating clinical aspects of care, and those developing the sociological, organisational, and theoretical domains in this area. This continuing divide is somewhat curious in the light of the following declaration from one of the architects of EBM himself, David Sackett:

> *'Evidence-based medicine (EBM) is the integration of best research evidence with clinical expertise and patient value... when these three elements are integrated, clinicians and patients form (an)... alliance which optimises clinical outcomes and quality of life...'* Sackett, 2000

In order to really understand this alliance, the research effort needs to be multidisciplinary, or even transdisciplinary, to address questions like: What is best evidence? What is the nature of values? How do they play out in organisational contexts? What kind of environments foster positive change? What kinds of outcomes matter, and to whom?

The series of studies presented in this volume offer a glimpse of some of the work that has been undertaken as part of the EU-funded COST network that was titled *'Childbirth Cultures, Concerns, and Consequences: Creating a dynamic EU framework for optimal maternity care'*. This network was set up precisely to catalyse interdisciplinary and transdisciplinary collaboration and to engender spread and reach of new paradigmatically goal-changing approaches to understanding how these aspects of evidence, values, practices and beliefs (among other things) interact, and how to implement change based on the findings to ensure that all learn from, and adapt to, the best.

Einstein is believed to have said '*Insanity is doing the same thing, over and over again, but expecting different results*'. The diverse studies presented in this volume offer insights that can help maternity care research and practice to move away from Einstein's trap of doing the same thing over and over again. They provide a new space in this field, underpinned by insights from multiple perspectives, and creating the potential to offer a new and exciting way forward for the future.

Soo Downe

August 7th 2016

Reference

Sackett DL (2000). *Evidence-Based Medicine: How to Practice and Teach EBM.* 2nd edn. Edinburgh; New York: Churchill Livingstone.

INTRODUCTION

Maternity care international perspectives: setting the scene

Edwin van Teijlingen, Lucy Frith and Sarah Church

Most women will become pregnant and have one or more babies in their life time. Although this is an almost universal experience, it is far from uniform. The expectations and experience of women are diverse, and the way that maternity care is organised in countries, regions or even smaller localities varies enormously. This book brings together an experienced team of health and social science researchers from different countries offering insights and potential lessons to be learnt about how maternity care can best be designed and delivered. It is, therefore, of interest for maternity care providers, managers, funders, policy-makers, and maternity pressure groups, as well as for women and their families.

This book has evolved out of the European COST Action IS0907 "Childbirth Cultures, Concerns and Consequences" (www.cost.eu/COST_Actions/isch/IS0907). The COST Action aimed to advance scientific knowledge about ways of improving maternity care provision and outcomes for mothers, babies and families. The four-year COST Action started in 2010 and ran until 2014. A total of 100 members from 26 countries were involved.

This chapter outlines the context for the collection, both practically and theoretically, and stresses the importance of conducting comparative research to find and generate the best possible evidence across a range of international childbirth practices, contexts, and issues. It sets out to establish the relevance of four different, but closely related, theoretical perspectives of health and healthcare which underpin the chapters within this book: (1) the concept of salutogenesis; (2) the medical/social model; (3) the humanisation of care; and (4) the notion of compassionate care. The first part of this chapter outlines each of these four approaches and their relevance to maternity services. It contextualises these debates in the light of the general shift towards a more risk-averse approach to childbirth globally, which is occurring at different rates across countries. The drivers to such changes also vary from country to country, but often the clinical, social and economic consequences are similar. These effects include unnecessary routine medicalisation of pregnancy and childbirth; increasing use of medical interventions/technology for individuals in response to population-based measures of risk; increasing hospitalisation for birth; dominance of the philosophy of one professional group over another, and of all professional groups over women and families using maternity care, resulting in distorted power relations/disempowerment; and, ultimately, loss of societal and individual belief in women's capacity (or even her moral right) to give birth physiologically.

Salutogenesis

One of the key theories used throughout this volume, is that of salutogenesis. The theory was developed by Aaron Antonovsky (1996), a medical sociologist. It hypothesises that everyone is on a continuum from full health to complete ill health (ultimately, death) and that individuals move along that continuum in different directions, and to different degrees, throughout their lives. The key underlying construct, the so-called 'sense of coherence', captures the extent to which someone believes that life is manageable, meaningful, and comprehensible, and the theory hypothesises that the more these three apply to an individual, the more likely they are to be at the health end of the continuum. When stressors and unexpected life events occur, the theory states that those with a higher sense of coherence will be more likely to be able to cope, and to maintain optimal health. When people experience a sense of coherence, Antonovsky argues that they would:

- Wish to and be motivated towards coping (meaningfulness)
- Believe that the challenge is understood (comprehensibility)
- Believe that the resources to cope are available to them (manageability).

The potential for salutogenesis to be applied to midwifery care is argued to begin with the aim of achieving optimal birth. Applying a salutogenic framework embraces the fundamental aim of empowering women to take control of childbirth. For this to take place, midwives need to adopt and apply a salutogenic approach. Browne and colleagues (2014), in their qualitative study on elements of salutogenesis, distilled three communication techniques used by midwives to promote a wellness focus in the antenatal period. These were: calm unhurriedness, speaking in wellness terms, and reassuring bodies. Similarly, Sinclair and Stockdale (2011) called for a radical change in midwifery education, in which salutogenic theory should be applied to shift the focus from a risk-averse curriculum to one which theoretically is more health promoting.

Medical/social model

The concept of the medical/social model is widely used in sociology to help analyse health-related phenomena such as obesity, alcohol misuse, shyness, infertility and disability. This in turn is linked to medicalisation, the process whereby diseases or conditions are no longer seen as a social issue or problem, but as primarily medical concerns. The concept of medicalisation theorises that society is more or less willingly allowing medicine to extend its power to more and more aspects of life (Conrad, 2005). When focused on pregnancy and childbirth the 'social' or 'midwifery' model is set against the 'medical' or 'obstetric' model (Van Teijlingen, 2005). Classically, the social model, when applied to maternity care, is associated with midwives, and is based on a philosophy which constructs pregnancy and birth as 'normal until proven otherwise'. In contrast, the medical model argues that 'childbirth is only safe in retrospect' (Van Teijlingen, 2005: 42). In other words, 'there appears to be an innate perception that birth is an event waiting to go wrong' (Lokugamage & Bourne, 2015: 164). To reduce this perceived risk, it is argued that birth is safer in hospital, with electronic fetal monitoring, and a range of interventions (e.g. forceps or caesarean sections), which are typically supervised by a doctor (Lothian, 2012: 46).

Anthropologist Robbie Davis-Floyd (1992) also identified these two opposing models of childbirth, but added a further nuance by juxtaposing the social construct of childbirth with what she termed the 'technocratic' model. More recently, it has been acknowledged that the two poles, however they are conceptualised, are archetypes that reflect professional projects, and not what either midwives or doctors actually do in practice (Renfrew et al, 2014). However, medical/technical risk-averse notions of pregnancy and birth do represent the dominant discourse in maternity care in most countries around the world, whatever their income status (MacKenzie-Bryers & van Teijlingen, 2010). One of the social consequences of the medical/technocratic model of childbirth becoming dominant, as Oakley (1980) argued, is the alienation of women from their bodies. More recently there have been concerns about disrespect and abuse of women and babies in institutional maternity care settings around the world (Bowser & Hill, 2010).

This leads us neatly to the next set of concepts used to identify or highlight changes in the social aspects of childbirth and maternity care.

Humanising maternity care

Mathew and Zadak (1997) remind us that the first attempts to humanise maternity care in the USA occurred in the 1940s with the birth of the 'prepared' or 'natural' childbirth movement. For Page (2001), reporting on the first Humanisation of Birth Conference held in Brazil, the key mechanism of humanisation is 'love between people, [as]… the basis for love in the family' (Page, 2001: S55). More recently, Todres and colleagues (2009) produced a theoretical framework based on the notion of humanising healthcare. They highlighted eight forms or processes of humanisation and dehumanisation in their work (see Table 1). This particular framework has been applied by others, for example, in the field of nursing (Hemingway *et al*, 2012) and public health (Hemingway, 2012). In this construction, humanisation works at an existential level. It relates to 'being' rather than 'doing'. Therefore, some claim that humanisation is more than providing holistic care, or recognising the 'wholeness' of the patient/person (Todres *et al*, 2009). If applied authentically, it can change our view of the world and our possibilities within that world. Humanisation therefore starts with the individual; not just the individual patient or service user, but also the individual service provider, whether part of the formal professional cadres or not. In this construction, if practitioners move towards the expression of humanised care, health services in general, and maternity services in particular, will change wholesale as a consequence.

Table 1:
Forms of humanising/dehumanising care (source: Todres *et al*, 2009)

FORMS OF HUMANISATION	FORMS OF DEHUMANISATION
• Insiderness	• Objectification
• Agency	• Passivity
• Uniqueness	• Homogenisation
• Togetherness	• Isolation
• Sense making	• Loss of meaning
• Personal journey	• Loss of personal journey
• Sense of place	• Dislocation
• Embodiment	• Reductionism

Compassionate care

Bowser and Hill (2010) were the first researchers to systematically explore the problem of disrespect and abuse in institutional maternity care settings around the world. They warn that poor staff behaviour is a serious deterrent to pregnant women and families using maternity care services (Bowser & Hill, 2010). Since they produced their report, there has been an explosion of interest in this area (Chadwick *et al*, 2014; Freedman & Kruk, 2014; Okafor *et al*, 2015).

On the flip side of disrespect and abuse, the area of compassionate and respectful care has been under researched until recently (Van Lerberghe *et al*, 2014). As an example of the newly emerging interest in this area, Clift and Steele (2015) conducted staff surveys incorporating notions of compassionate care in a North London Integrated Care Organisation. From their qualitative analysis of 218 responses to the survey they proposed a model of the concept of compassion. They concluded that the key process that made compassion 'happen' was communication: 'Compassion begins with an observation, and then communication takes place involving listening and helping' (Clift & Steele, 2015: 23).

In common with other areas of healthcare, poor communication between staff and maternity users, poor or inadequate information, and negative attitudes and behaviours of maternity staff are linked to new mothers' negative feelings such as fear, anger, disappointment, stress, guilt and feeling inadequate (Barker *et al*, 2005: 315). Cooper (2015: 57) links compassion to the notion of courage, as she argues that maternity care providers struggle in their ability to provide compassionate care. These challenges include the circumstances in which they work, the organisational climate in their workplace, and their role and position in the occupational hierarchy. Moreover, Campling (2015: 19) notes that health workers themselves need to be supported and made to feel that they are valued, they 'need to be listened to, nurtured, developed and encouraged if they are to enact the qualities required to provide sensitive, compassionate maternity care.'

Indeed, moving towards a maternity service that is based on care and compassion needs to start with student education. As Lokugamage and Bourne (2015: 166) observe, 'students will not see kindness, dignity and respect unless they have the opportunity to witness it and see it modelled within the care and their families.'

Bringing it together

This book therefore offers an exploration of a new set of theories to help explain the nature of maternity care provision across Europe and beyond. The aim is to examine the nature of these theories, and to demonstrate how they can be applied to a range of practical situations across a number of different countries.

The final section of this chapter describes how these aims are met, chapter by chapter.

In Chapter 2, Bengt Lindström, Marie Berg, Claudia Meier Magistretti, Mercedes Perez-Botella and Soo Downe examine the potential for salutogenic theory as a framework for maternity care research and practice. By drawing on existing evidence, it is shown that salutogenesis can complement medicine and technology by being implemented as a health-related maternity care practice. The authors present evidence of the value of salutogenic analysis and its use as a lens to investigate aspects within maternity care. Gaps in current knowledge are considered and a research programme for further work is proposed.

In Chapter 3, Helga Gottfreðsdóttir, Marianne Nieuwenhuijze and Lucy Frith address the use of complexity theory to reflect on the implementation process of antenatal screening and diagnosis in three countries – Iceland, the Netherlands and the United Kingdom. By applying the taxonomy of complexity theory, the authors present an analysis of the nature of complexity in the development of fetal screening services. Interconnectivity, open boundaries and self-organisation were reported to have a strong influence on the implementation of fetal screening across the three countries.

In Chapter 4, Valerie Smith, Cecily Begley, Mechthild M. Gross and Declan Devane discuss the concept of care outcomes in health conditions in maternity care research and their use in systematic reviews, trials and other studies. The authors consider the development and rationale for the use of an agreed set of outcomes, known as 'core outcome sets' (COS), in maternity care practice and research as a means by which to address outcome variation and outcome reporting bias.

In Chapter 5, Jette Aaroe Clausen and Mário JDS Santos explore the use of in-labour ethnography as a means of examining what goes beyond the taken-for-granted understandings of everyday practice. Whilst the authors reflect on both the productive and problematic features of in-labour ethnography, by reflecting on their own experiences they argue the merits of the approach to illuminate social phenomena which would otherwise be hidden or be inaccessible to other researchers.

In Chapter 6, Karin Minnie and Christa van der Walt discuss the role of a working group on knowledge transfer in a COST action study. The authors discuss the challenges of planning the knowledge transfer process for a multidisciplinary international research project and begin with a discussion of the multiplicity of terms used to describe the process. They discuss a framework for knowledge transfer and suggest that researchers need to identify an appropriate knowledge transfer strategy during the proposal stage and review it during the course of the study.

In Chapter 7, Berit Viken, Marie-Clare Balaam and Anne Lyberg examine the position of migrant women and maternity care in Europe from a salutogenic perspective. They consider the ways in which a salutogenic approach can enhance understanding of the maternity needs and experiences of women who migrate to Europe. Using case studies from research work in Norway, they assert that a salutogenic approach would be useful to recognise more fully the strengths, resilience and coping strategies of these women as they navigate pregnancy and motherhood in their new countries.

In Chapter 8, Sarah Church and Olga Gouni consider some of the key issues which relate to the migration of midwives. Against the background of limited literature, the authors explore the process and experience of acculturation using a salutogenic model and consider the wider issues of workforce integration. This chapter concludes with a focus on the development of the global midwife and considers some of the challenges and opportunities for this role.

In Chapter 9, Christa van der Walt and Karin Minnie discuss their involvement in the development and implementation of the Africa Maternal-Child Health Nurse Leadership Academy (MCHNLA). They outline the need for strong leaders and consider some of the challenges faced by midwives in transforming healthcare services. Using a theoretical framework, they demonstrate how leadership can be learned within a mentorship leadership experience using a triad of mentee, mentor and faculty consultant. They conclude that leadership development can be a vehicle for the transformation of maternal-child health and maternity services provision.

In Chapter 10, Ans Luyben, Claudia Meier Magistretti, Barbara Kaiser, Iréne Maffi and Annette Kuhn reflect on their participation and contribution to the first COST Action from 2010 to 2014. The authors discuss how being an active group within the COST Action enabled the formation of maternity care research in Switzerland. Within their reflection, they focus on their experience of undertaking three core studies, and discuss how this work has contributed to national knowledge about maternity care and to the COST Action.

In the final chapter, Valerie Smith, Cecily Begley and Declan Devane present an in-depth discussion and analysis of the first systematic review of women's views, experiences and perceptions of fetal heart rate monitoring during labour. Against the background of insufficient high-quality evidence to support the use of electronic fetal monitoring in low-risk pregnancies, the findings of the review present useful insights into the use and choice of fetal heart rate monitoring methods, and present clinical decision makers with areas to consider when implementing policy and practice changes.

References

Antonovsky A (1996). The salutogenic model as a theory to guide health promotion. *Health Prom Intl* 11(1): 11-18.

Barker SR, Precilla YL, Henshaw CA & Tree J (2005). "I felt as though I'd been in jail": Women's experiences of maternity care in labour, delivery and the immediate postpartum. *J Feminism Psychol* 15(3): 315–342.

Bowser D & Hill K (2010). *Exploring Evidence for Disrespect and Abuse in Facility-Based Childbirth: Report of a Landscape Analysis. USAID-TRAction Project.* [online]. Harvard, MA.: Harvard School of Public Health, University Research Co., LLC. Available from: http://xa.yimg.com/kq/groups/17806146/113687991/name/Exploring+Evidence+for+Disrespect+and+Abuse+in+Facility-Based+Childbirth+Report.pdf

Browne J, O'Brien M, Taylor J, Bowman R & Davis D (2014). 'You've got it within you': the political act of keeping a wellness focus in the antenatal time. *Midwifery* 30(4): 420-426.

Campling P (2015). Putting relationships at the heart of maternity care. In: Downe S and Byrom S (eds). *The Roar Behind the Silence.* London: Pinter and Martin, pp15-20.

Chadwick RJ, Cooper D & Harries J (2014). Narratives of distress about birth in South African public maternity settings: A qualitative study. *Midwifery* 30: 862–868.

Clift M & Steele S (2015). Compassion in hospital care staff: what they think it is, what gets in its way, and how to enhance it. In: Downe S. and Byrom S (eds). *The Roar Behind the Silence.* London: Pinter and Martin, pp21-26.

Conrad P (2005). The shifting engines of medicalization. *J Health Soc Behav* 46: 3-13.

Cooper T (2015). Promoting normal birth: courage through compassion. In: Downe S and Byrom S (eds). *The Roar Behind the Silence. London*: Pinter and Martin, pp57-61.

Davis-Floyd R (1992). *Birth as an American Rite of Passage.* Berkeley: University of California Press.

Freedman LP & Kruk ME (2014). Disrespect and abuse of women in childbirth: challenging the global quality and accountability agendas. *Lancet* 384 (9948): e42–e44.

Hemingway A (2012). Can humanisation theory contribute to the philosophical debate in public health? *Public Health* 126: 448-453.

Hemingway A, Scammell J & Heaslip V (2012). Humanising nursing care: a theoretical model. *Nursing Times* 108(40): 26-227.

Lokugamage A & Bourne T (2015). They don't know what they don't know. In: Downe S & Byrom S (eds). *The Roar Behind the Silence.* London: Pinter and Martin, pp162-167.

Lothian JA (2012). Risk, safety, and choice in childbirth. *J Perinat Educ* 21(1): 45-47.

MacKenzie Bryers H & Van Teijlingen E (2010). Risk, theory, social & medical models: a critical analysis of the concept of risk in maternity care. *Midwifery* 26(5): 488-496.

Mathew JJ & Zadak K (1997). The alternative birth movement in the United States: History and current status. In: Apple RD, Golden J (eds). *Mothers and Motherhood: Readings in American History.* Columbus, Ohio: Ohio State University Press, pp278-292.

Nicholls L & Webb C (2006). What makes a good midwife? Methodologically diverse research. *J Advanc Nurs* 56(4): 414-429.

Oakley A (1980). *Women Confined. Towards a Sociology of Childbirth.* Oxford: Martin Robertson.

Okafor I, Ugwu EO & Obi SN (2015). Disrespect and abuse during facility-based childbirth in a low-income country. *Int J Gynaecol Obstet* 128 110–113.

Page L (2001). The humanization of birth. *Int J Gynecol Obstetr* 75: S55-58.

Renfrew MJ, McFadden A, Bastos MH et al (2014). Midwifery and quality care: findings from a new evidence-informed framework for maternal and newborn care. *Lancet* Sep 20; 384(9948): 1129-1145.

Sinclair M & Stockdale J (2011). Achieving optimal birth using salutogenesis in routine antenatal education. *Evidence Based Midwifery* 9: 75.

Todres L, Galvin, K & Holloway I (2009). The humanization of healthcare: a value framework for qualitative research. *Int J Qual Stud Health Well-being* 4(2): 68-77.

Van Lerberghe W, Matthews Z, Achadi E *et al* (2014). Country experience with strengthening of health systems and deployment of midwives in countries with high maternal mortality. *Lancet* 384: 1215-1225.

Van Teijlingen E (2005). A critical analysis of the medical model as used in the study of pregnancy and childbirth. *Sociological Research Online* 10(2).

CHAPTER 1

The salutogenic approach to maternity care: from theory to practice and research

Bengt Lindström, Marie Berg, Claudia Meier Magistretti, Mercedes Perez-Botella and Soo Downe

Introduction

For most of recorded history, pregnancy and childbirth for individual women has been understood as a largely normative psychosocial and physiological event, best left to the becoming-mother and her intimate family, often with the support of experienced lay attendants, usually local women. However, at the population level, the maternity episode is also framed sociologically, usually with specific rituals, prohibitions and rights (Jordan & Davis-Floyd, 1993; Davis-Floyd, 2004). Since the early 1970s, researchers and philosophers working in this area have noted a cross-cultural shift in these societal norms, which has been attributed variously to medicalisation, technocracy, scientific bureaucracy, modernist risk aversion, super-valuation of a surveillance culture, and/or patriarchy (Arney, 1982; Arms, 1997; Ehrenreich & English, 2005; Ehrenreich & English, 2010). Whatever the underlying driver for this global shift, the consequence is that childbirth is now mainly seen as a risky event, only normal (healthy) in retrospect, and only safeguarded by routine medical-technical monitoring.

This shift in societal perception has also created a professional division between the two disciplines that are most often at the front line of maternity care, midwifery and obstetrics. The underlying tenets of midwifery continue to promote the physiology of pregnancy, labour and the postpartum period (Renfrew *et al*, 2014). Those of obstetrics are, in contrast, more closely aligned to a 'just in case' philosophy where the health of the mother and the baby is not assumed (Arney, 1982). Individual practitioners in both disciplines are, however, subject to the general post-modernist risk aversion that characterises late-modernist societies (Giddens, 1991; Beck, 1992). This means that, despite their professional belief systems, many qualified midwives are practising in highly technical environments where trust in physiological labour and birth is overshadowed by risk-averse systems and behaviours, and disease-focused rules and protocols.

It is now well-accepted that the dominant way of doing birth across the world has adverse consequences for women, babies, families, and the professionals who attend them, and that it is not sustainable in the long run (Moynihan, Heneghan & Godlee, 2013). One way of challenging the hegemony of risk-averse maternity care is to re-establish a positive health perspective. This process can be supported by a theory on how health in its origin is created and promoted. One promising approach is salutogenesis as first presented by Aaron Antonovsky (Antonovsky, 1979, 1987; Lindström & Ericsson, 2010). This chapter will explore how salutogenesis can be implemented as a health-related maternity care practice and as a complement to medicine and technology. The basic priniciples of salutogenesis theory are presented, followed by an exploration of the scientific evidence for its explanatory power, and why it may be important for maternity care. The chapter concludes with an exploration of gaps in the current knowledge base in this area, and the consequent future challenges for stakeholders, including service providers, and researchers.

What is the salutogenic framework?

The salutogenic framework was developed by the medical sociologist Aaron Antonovsky in the late 1970s as part of his interest in stress (Antonovsky, 1979; 1987). His developing interest in this area started with an epidemiological study on the effects of menopause on women who had undergone extreme stressful life events, including some who had survived the Holocaust (Antonovsky, 1979). As anticipated, most of these women found life much more stressful than women who had not experienced such life events (control group women). However, against Antonovsky's expectation, a small group of the Holocaust survivors recorded similar levels of day-to-day stress as those in the control group. Antonovsky was absorbed by how it was at all possible for the women from the Holocaust to be able to carry on with daily life including to love, and to have positive social relationships with children, families, and work colleagues. This led Antonovsky to pose the question: 'What creates health?' This question became a turning point for the creation of a new paradigm – the health-promotive movement.

In subsequent studies, Antonovsky and his colleages analysed a large number of narratives from people who had survived the Holocaust, and still maintained good health and led satisfying lives. They found common patterns in the narratives that led to salutogenesis. Conceptually, salutogenesis is defined as a process through which the individual strives to move towards the health end of the ease / dis-ease continuum (Antonovsky, 1993). The direction of this movement towards health and wellbeing, even in the presence of adverse life events, is supported by 'generalised resistance resources' (GRR) that are available in moments of stress. The GRRs include both internal resources, such as knowledge and attitudes, and external ones, such as social support and access to essential societal characteristics such as security and peace. The capacity to use these resources frames a consistent global orientation, which expresses a 'sense of coherence' (SOC). This includes three central dimensions: comprehensibility, manageability and meaningfulness. A basic presupposition for the theory is that people with a strong sense of coherence believe that life events, even stressful ones, are generally understandable and explicable challenges worthy of investment and engagement, and they are manageable by the resources available to a person (Antonovsky, 1987). Based on this, Antonovsky constructed an instrument, the Orientation to Life Questionnaire, or the SOC scale as it is more usually known as (Antonovsky, 1987). The theory was that individuals, groups and societies with a stronger sense of coherence experience better health and wellbeing over time.

Over the last 25 years, this theory has been tested in a range of cultural settings around the world, and it appears to have a strong empirical basis (Eriksson & Lindström, 2006; Eriksson & Lindström, 2007). Generally, a strong sense of coherence is associated with reduced anxiety, depression, burnout and hopelessness, and strongly and positively related to health resources such as optimism, hardiness, control, and coping. A strong sense of coherence can generally predict good health and quality of life from childhood to adulthood, and can specifically predict the risk of mental health issues: the stronger the sense of coherence, the fewer the symptoms of mental illnesses (Lindstrom & Eriksson, 2010). In summary, Antonovsky's salutogenic theory presents health as a process of becoming over the life course. It sees people as active participating subjects in the process of their lives; the development of a strong sense of coherence is a lifelong process (Lindström & Eriksson, 2011). The theory also provides a challenge to the current emphasis on ill health in maternity care.

Why a salutogenic framework for maternity care?

Evidence is beginning to emerge that routine 'just in case' interventions in pregnancy and childbirth that are applied to whole populations may be interrupting healthy adaptive processes that are essential for the wellbeing of the mother and baby, in both the short and longer term (Dahlen *et al*, 2013). This suggests that the optimum approach should be a focus on promoting health, wellbeing and a strong sense of coherence, rather than undermining these important phenomena with routine risk-averse pharmacological and technical interventions, unless there is a strong and evident clinical need for them. Psychosocially, a supportive family environment in childhood enhances the level and heritability of sense of coherence in early adulthood (Silventoinen *et al*, 2014).

Children's and adolescents' health, in addition to mothers´ and parents´ ability to cope with children's life events, illnesses or disabilities, is strongly and positively related to a strong sense of coherence (Einav, Levi & Margalit, 2012; Hedov, Anneren & Wikblad, 2002; Pozo Cabanillas *et al*, 2006; Svavarsdottir, McCubbin & Kane, 2000; Schmitt *et al*, 2008). Few, but similar, findings exist for single-parent mothers, whose demoralisation is negatively associated with their sense of coherence (Soskolne, 2001). In parents, a strong sense of coherence influences the ability to cope with (chronic) illness or disability of their children (Olsson & Hwang, 2008; Schmitt *et al*, 2008). A parent's sense of coherence is also directly correlated with children's psychosomatic complaints – if the latter are lower, the former scores are high.

For pregnancy and birth, results show that a strong sense of coherence is correlated with fewer birth complications (Oz *et al*, 2009) and has a moderating effect on anticipated and supported stress during pregnancy (Hibino *et al*, 2009). Women with a strong sense of coherence have demonstrated increased coping with emergency caesarean sections and show less post-traumatic symptoms after the event (Tham, Chistensson & Ryding, 2007). They quit smoking in pregnancy more often (Abrahamsson & Ejlertsson, 2002), and they tend to choose natural birth instead of planned caesarean sections or other technical interventions (Hellmers &

Schuecking, 2008). A strong connection with the sense of coherence has been measured empirically, mainly in correlation with positive outcome variables such as higher rates of breastfeeding, higher satisfaction with care or birth experience, better perceived control during birth, easier bonding with the baby, higher maternal self-esteem and parental confidence or with less negative perception of pain (Perrez-Botella *et al*, 2014).

Although the relevance of salutogenesis has been discussed for the postnatal period and very early life also, the sense of coherence itself, its development and changes, have not yet been systematically investigated in the transition from birth to the period of early motherhood. Most of the discussion reveals conceptual or general considerations only, and there are few published empirical research studies undertaken in the postnatal period and in the first year after birth (Perez-Botella *et al*, 2014). Thomson and Dykes (2011) showed that a strong sense of coherence in mothers in the early postnatal period is associated with increased success in breastfeeding. Earlier studies found low postpartum depression rates and better wellbeing after birth associated with a stronger sense of coherence (Hellmers, Geburtsmodus & Wohlbefinden, 2005). Other authors stated that the maternal sense of coherence contributes significantly to children's secure attachment and to various socio-emotional adjustment measures (Al-Yagon, 2008) as well as to family cohesion generally (Einav, Levi & Margalit, 2012).

Little is known yet about factors influencing a strong sense of coherence in mothers during the first year after childbirth, though some evidence shows that high-quality health services might be beneficial for a mother's sense of coherence, and even that such services might compensate for a lack of strong neighbourhood-networks (Lagerberg, Magnusson & Sundelin, 2011). Future research in this field is important, since high-quality care in (early) childhood is known to foster a strong sense of coherence in adulthood (Hakanen, Feldt & Leskinen, 2007). Eickhorst *et al* (2010) included the measurement of sense of coherence in their investigation of parents participating in an early life care programme. Their findings revealed higher SOC scores in fathers than in mothers of families with psychosocial stress. These findings confirm the results of studies comparing mothers' and fathers' sense of coherence that showed higher scores on fathers' SOC in both families with healthy as well as with disabled or chronically ill children (Grøholt *et al*, 2003; Olsson & Hwang, 2002; Sivberg, 2002; Svavarsdottir, McCubbin & Kane, 2000).

This evidence, albeit presently limited, demonstrates that mothers and/or fathers with a strong sense of coherence in the postnatal period may have a positive influence on their children's sense of coherence in the longer term. However, there is very little research on if and how the maternal/paternal sense of coherence can be directly reinforced and/or undermined by their experiences during pregnancy, childbirth and the postpartum period. Originally, the sense of coherence was assumed to be a stable orientation in life, after early adulthood (Antonovsky, 1987; Sagy & Antonovsky, 2000; Abrahamsson & Ejlertsson, 2002; Oz *et al*, 2009). Although this assumption has been confirmed in some research (e.g. Kivimaki *et al*, 2000; Hakanen, Feldt & Leskinen, 2007), changes in the sense of coherence later in life have also been demonstrated (Johansson *et al*, 2009). One study has reported a strengthened sense of coherence due to interventions in the area of mental health (Jönsson *et al*, 2011). Antonovsky himself acknowledged that his early assumption that the sense of coherence is unlikely to change after the age of about 30 might be flawed, since he made this assumption by focusing on people with a strong sense of coherence. More recent work has revealed that those with lower values are more susceptible to changes of an upward nature in the presence of a seminal event with positive connotations (Hakanen, Feldt & Leskinen, 2007). This is crucially important in relation to maternity populations, firstly because having children past the third decade of life is not uncommon, and, secondly, because childbirth is a major event in a woman's life with high potential to influence sense of coherence levels.

Sjostrom and colleagues (Sjostrom, Langius-Eklof & Hjertberg, 2004) found a slight decline in the sense of coherence in mothers towards the end of pregnancy, but no improvement in the sense of coherence after birth. In contrast, more recent work has found that birth and parenthood could lead to a remarkable increase in the sense of coherence in mothers (Röhl & Schücking, 2006; Habroe & Schmidt, 2007). Specific data for fathers' changes in the sense of coherence do not exist in this context, but research on self-efficacy indicates an increase in fathers' parenting self-efficacy and satisfaction in the period of transition to parenthood when participating in an early life care programme for fathers (Hudson *et al*, 2003).

Discussion

The recent *Lancet* series on midwifery has conceptualised midwifery as:

> *'Skilled, knowledgeable and compassionate care for childbearing women, newborn infants and families across the continuum throughout pre-pregnancy, pregnancy, birth, postpartum and the early weeks of life. Core*

> *characteristics include optimising normal biological, psychological, social, and cultural processes of reproduction and early life, timely prevention and management of complications, consultation with and referral to other services, respecting women's individual circumstances and views, and working in partnership with women to strengthen women's own capabilities to care for themselves and their families.'* (Renfrew *et al*, 2014, p3)

This definition allows for the inclusion of professionals other than midwives, and skilled and experienced lay providers of supportive maternity care. The series also presents a Quality Maternity and Newborn Care framework (Renfrew *et al*, 2014) that clearly prioritises a salutogenic-type approach, in which the majority of women and babies are seen as healthy, and where the main job of caregivers is to support and to reinforce the healthy end of the salutogenic continuum.

These high-level publications indicate that the mood is changing in maternity care around the world. It is increasingly evident that risk-averse, just-in-case maternity systems are associated with adverse effects for mothers, babies and families, and that they are too expensive for societies to maintain. The evidence summarised in this chapter suggests that, beyond a general turn to thinking about wellbeing rather than about risk, the components of salutogenic theory might lend themsleves to rigorous scientific research in this area. Along with other new ways of thinking, such as those generated by complexity theory (Downe & McCourt, 2008), realist research advocates (Pawson *et al*, 2005) and by groups such as the *BMJ*'s 'Too Much Medicine' campaign (Moynihan, Heneghan & Godlee, 2013) and its international associates, salutogenesis theory offers an exciting new avenue for maternity care research and practice. Integration of some of these new, health-focused ways of conceptualising pregnancy and childbirth is beginning to be evidenced in curriculum development in both midwifery and obstetrics (Downe, 2010; Feinland & Sankey, 2008) and in healthcare provision (Rotundo, 2011; Tilden *et al*, 2014; Sandall *et al*, 2016; Hodnett *et al*, 2010). A possible research programme is set out in the next section.

Research gaps

The overview presented in this chapter demonstrates a lack of systematic investigation into the nature of pregnancy, childbirth and the postpartum period, and into the provision of maternity care, from a salutogenic orientation. Specific areas for research include:

- The correlates and influencing factors of a weak or strong sense of coherence during pregnancy, childbirth and early mothering, and especially the effects of marital and social support, psychological and socioeconomic determinants, and a positive experience with minimal external clinical and/or pharmacological interventions, in healthy as well as in vulnerable groups of women;
- The degree to which a particularly weak or a particularly strong sense of coherence might predict a physically, emotionally and psychosocially healthy maternity episode, for mother, baby and family;
- The influence of pregnancy, intrapartum and postnatal experiences on changes in the sense of coherence between early pregnancy and the end of the postpartum period;
- The differential effects, if any, of physiologically healthy and/or emotionally positive childbirth and early mothering (including breastfeeding) on SOC levels for postnatal women, when compared to similar women who have experienced routine interventions/negative experiences.

Conclusion

It is widely accepted that there are adverse maternal, neonatal and familial effects of routine unnecessary interventions in pregnancy, childbirth and the postnatal period. Despite this, rates of such interventions continue to rise. The inability to reverse this trend may be partially explained by a persistent focus on risk aversion in maternity care. Salutogenic theory offers an alternative and potentially powerful lens through which to understand the value of non-intervention unless it is absolutely necessary. This chapter has presented evidence for the value of salutogenic analysis in fields beyond maternity care, and has summarised the results of the small number of studies conducted to date within the pregnancy, childbirth and postnatal period. The summary suggests that there is significant potential for research in this area to be the basis for change in maternity care provision. The research topics proposed above offer a guide for a future research programme in this area.

References

Abrahamsson A & Ejlertsson GA (2002). Salutogenic perspective could be of practical relevance for the prevention of smoking amongst pregnant women. *Midwifery* 18: 323-331.

Al-Yagon M (2008). Maternal personal resources and children's socioemotional and behavioural adjustment. *Child Psychiatry Hum Develop* 39(3): 283-298.

Antonovsky A (1993). *The salutogenic approach to aging*. Lecture held in Berkeley, January 21, 1993.

Antonovsky A (1987). *Unraveling the Mystery of Health: How People Manage Stress and Stay Well*. San Francisco: Jossey-Bass.

Antonovsky A (1979). *Health, Stress and Coping*. San Francisco: Jossey-Bass.

Arms S (1997). *Immaculate Deception II: Myth, Magic and Birth*. Berkeley, California: Celestial Arts.

Arney WR (1982). *Power and the Profession of Obstetrics*. Chicago: University Chicago Press.

Beck U (1992). *Risk Society: Towards a New Modernity*. New Delhi: Sage.

Dahlen HG, Kennedy HP, Anderson CM, Bell AF, Clark A, Foureur M, Ohm JE, Shearman AM, Taylor JY, Wright ML & Downe S (2013). The EPIIC hypothesis: intrapartum effects on the neonatal epigenome and consequent health outcomes. *Med Hypotheses* 280(5):656-662.

Davis-Floyd R (2004). *Birth as an American Rite of Passage*. 2nd edn. University of California Press.

Downe S (2010). Beyond evidence-based medicine: complexity, and stories of maternity care. *J Eval Clin Prac* 16(1): 232-237.

Downe S & McCourt C (2008). From being to becoming: reconstructing childbirth knowledges. In: Downe S (ed). *Normal Birth: Evidence and Debate*. 2nd edn. Oxford: Elsevier.

Ehrenreich B & English D (2010). *Witches, Midwives and Nurses: A History of Women Healers*. 2nd edn. The City University of New York, Feminist Press.

Ehrenreich B & English D (2005). *For Her Own Good: Two Centuries of the Experts' Advice to Women*. New York: Anchor Books.

Eickhorst A, Schweyer D, Köhler H, Jelen-Mauboussin A, Kunz E, Sidor A & Cierpka M (2010). Elterliche Feinfühligkeit bei Müttern und Vätern mit psychosozialen Belastungen. *Bundesgesundheitsblatt* 53:1126-1133.

Einav M, Levi U & Margalit M (2012). Mothers' coping and hope in early intervention. *Eur J Spec Needs Educ* 27(3): 265-279.

Eriksson M & Lindstrom B (2007). Antonovsky's sense of coherence scale and the relationship with quality of life: a systematic review. *J Epidemiol Community Health* 61: 938-944.

Eriksson M & Lindstrom B (2006). Antonovsky's sense of coherence scale and the relation with health: a systematic review. *J Epidemiol Community Health* 60: 376-381.

Feinland JB & Sankey HZ (2008). The obstetrics team: midwives teaching residents and medical students on the labor and delivery unit. *J Midwifery Womens Health* 253(4): 376-380.

Giddens A (1991). *Modernity and Self-Identity. Self and Society in the Late Modern Age*. Cambridge: Polity Press – Blackwell Publishing.

Grøholt E-K, Stigum H, Nordhagen R & Köhler L (2003). Is parental sense of coherence associated with child health? *Eur J Public Health* 13(3): 195-201.

Habroe M & Schmidt L (2007). Does childbirth after fertility treatment influence SOC? A longitudinal study of 1934 men and women. *Acta Obstet Gynecol Scand* 86(10): 1215-1221.

Hakanen JJ, Feldt T & Leskinen E (2007). Change and stability of sense of coherence in adulthood: Longitudinal evidence from the Healthy Child study. *J Res Pers* 41(3): 602-661.

Hedov G, Annerén G & Wikblad K (2002). Swedish parents of children with Down's syndrome. Parental stress and sense of coherence in relation to employment rate and time spent in child care. *Scand J Caring Sci* 16: 424-430.

Hellmers C & Schuecking B (2008). Primiparae's well-being before and after birth and relationship with preferred and actual mode of birth in Germany and the USA. *J Reprod Infant Psychol* 26(4): 351-372.

Hellmers C (2005). Geburtsmodus und Wohlbefinden. Eine prospektive Untersuchung an Erstgebärenden unter besonderer Berücksichtigung des (Wunsch-)Kaiserschnittes. [Birth mode and well-being. A prospective study on primiparae with special regard to caesarean section wish.] Aachen: Shaker Verlag.

Hibino Y, Takaki J, Kambayashi Y, Hitomi Y, Sakai A, Sekizuka N, Ogino K & Nakamura H (2009). Health impact of disaster-related stress on pregnant women living in the affected area of the Noto Peninsula earthquake in Japan. *Psychiatry Clin Neurosci* 63(1):107-115.

Hodnett ED, Downe S, Walsh D & Weston J (2010). Alternative versus conventional institutional settings for birth. *Cochrane Database of Systematic Reviews* 9: CD000012.

Hudson DB, Campbell-Grossman C, Fleck MO, Elek SM & Shipman A (2003). Effects of the New Fathers Network on first-time fathers' parenting self efficacy and parenting satisfaction during the transition to parenthood. *Compr Pediatr Nurs* 26(4): 217-229.

Johansson M, Adolfsson A, Berg M, Francis J, Hogström L, Janson PO, Sogn J & Hellström AL (2009). Quality of life for couples 4-5.5 years after unsuccessful IVF treatment. *Acta Obstet Gynecol Scand* 88: 291-300.

Jönsson PD, Wijk H, Danielson E & Skärsäter I (2011). Outcomes of an educational intervention for the family of a person with bipolar disorder: a 2-year follow-up study. *J Psychiatr Ment Health Nurs* 18: 333-341

Jordan B & Davis-Floyd R. *Birth in Four Cultures: A Crosscultural Investigation of Childbirth in Yucatan, Holland, Sweden and the United States.* Waveland Press.

Kivimaki M, Feldt T, Vahtera J & Nurmi JE (2000). Sense of coherence and health: evidence from two cross-lagged longitudinal samples. *Soc Sci Med* 50(4): 583-597.

Lagerberg D, Magnusson M & Sundelin C (2011). Child health and maternal stress: does neighbourhood status matter? *Int J Adolesc Med Health* 23(1): 19-25.

Lindström & Eriksson M (2011). From health education to healthy learning: Implementing salutogenesis in educational science. *Scand J Public Health* 39: 85-92.

Lindström B & Eriksson M (2010). *The Hitchhiker's Guide to Salutogenesis: Salutogenic Pathways to Health Promotion.* Helsinki: Folkhälsan Press.

Moynihan R, Heneghan C & Godlee F (2013). Too much medicine: from evidence to action. *BMJ* 347: f7141.

Olsson MB & Hwang CP (2008). Socioeconomic and psychological variables as risk and protective factors for parental well-being in families of children with intellectual disabilities. *J Intellect Disabil Res* 52(12): 1102-1113.

Olsson MB & Hwang CP (2002). Sense of coherence in parents of children with different developmental disabilities. *J Intellect Disabil Res* 46(7): 548-559.

Oz Y, Sarid O, Peleg R & Sheiner E (2009). Sense of coherence predicts uncomplicated delivery: a prospective observational study. *J Psychosom Obstet Gynecol* 30(1): 29-33.

Pawson R, Greenhalgh T, Harvey G & Walshe K (2005). Realist review – a new method of systematic review designed for complex policy interventions. *J Health Serv Res Policy* 10(suppl 1): 21-34.

Perez-Botella M, Downe S, Meier Magistretti C, Lindstrom B & Berg M (2014). The use of salutogenesis theory in empirical studies of maternity care for healthy mothers and babies. *Sex Reprod Healthc* 6(1):33-9.

Pozo Cabanillas P, Sarria Sanchez E & Mendez Zaballos L (2006). Stress in mothers of individuals with autistic spectrum disorders. *Psicothema* 18(3): 342-347.

Renfrew MJ, McFadden A, Bastos MH, Campbell J, Channon AA, Cheung NF, Delage D, Downe SM, Kennedy HP, Malata A, McCormick F, Wick L & Declercq E (2014). Midwifery and quality care: findings from a new evidence-informed maternity care framework. *Lancet* 384(9948): 1129-1145.

Röhl S & Schücking B (2006). Veränderungen des Kohärenzgefühls nach der Geburt. Eine prospektive Stuide bei Frauen mit stationär behandelter vorzeitiger Wehentätigkeit. *Psychotherapie, Psychosomatik, Medizinische Psychologie* 56-A78.

Rotundo G (2011). Centering pregnancy: the benefits of group prenatal care. *Nurs Womens Health* 15(6): 208-217.

Sandall J, Soltani H, Gates S, Shennan A & Devane D (2016). Midwife-led continuity models versus other models of care for childbearing women. *Cochrane Database of Systematic Reviews* 8: CD004667.

Sagy S & Antonovsky H (2000). The development of the sense of coherence: a retrospective study of early life experiences in the family. *Int J Aging Hum Dev* 51(2): 155-166.

Schmitt F, Santalahti P, Saarelainen S, Savonlahti E, Romer G & Piha J (2008). Cancer families with children: factors associated with family functioning – a comparative study in Finland. *Psychooncology* 17(4):363-372.

Silventoinen H, Voanen SM, Vuksimaa E & Rose RJ (2014). A supportive family environment in childhood enhances the level and heritability of sense of coherence in early adulthood. *Soc Psychiatry Psychiatr Epidemiol* 49(12): 1951-1960.

Sivberg B (2002). Coping strategies and parental attitudes. A comparison of parents with children with autistic spectrum disorders and parents with non-autistic children. *Int J Circumpolar Health* 61(suppl 2): 36-35.

Sjostrom H, Langius-Eklof A & Hjertberg R (2004). Well-being and sense of coherence during pregnancy. *Acta Obstet Gynecol Scand* 83(12):1112-1118.

Soskolne V (2001). Single parenthood, occupational drift and psychological distress among immigrant women from the former Soviet Union in Israel. *Women Health* 33(3-4): 67-84.

Svavarsdottir EK, McCubbin MA & Kane JH (2000). Well-being of parents of young children with asthma. *Res Nurs Health* 23(5): 346-358.

Tham V, Christensson K & Ryding EL (2007). SOC and symptoms of post-traumatic stress after emergency CS. *Acta Obstet Gynecol Scand* 86(9):1090-1096.

Thomson G & Dykes F (2011). Women's sense of coherence related to their infant feeding experience. *Matern Child Nutr* 7(2): 160-174.

Tilden EL, Hersh SR, Emeis CL, Weinstein SR & Caughey AB (2014). Group prenatal care: review of outcomes and recommendations for model implementation. *Obstet Gynecol Surv* 69(1): 46-55.

CHAPTER 2

Fetal screening in three countries from a complexity theory perspective

Helga Gottfreðsdóttir, Marianne Nieuwenhuijze and Lucy Frith

Maternity care services are constantly challenged by stakeholders to optimise their provision. Individual care users, consumer organisations, staff, researchers, policy makers, professional organisations, media, insurance companies, politicians and governments will try and provoke change at different levels. There is pressure on these services to provide high-quality care, safety, adequate working conditions, up-to-date technology and cost-effective treatment and interventions. At the same time, legal and ethical issues, such as equal access and fair division of resources, also require consideration. To address these demands, maternity care services need to be able to adapt dynamically and function as complex adaptive systems (Committee on Quality Health Care in America, Institute of Medicine, 2001; Plsek & Greenhalgh, 2001).

According to Cillers (1998) a complex adaptive system is characterised as a non-linear system. Maternity care is complex because of the great number of interconnections between different agents within and among different care organisations. Maternity care services are adaptive because staff and care users have the capacity to learn and change their behaviour. How this behaviour changes is not always predictable, and contributes to variation in the delivery of care (Committee on Quality Health Care in America, Institute of Medicine, 2001). The provision of similar healthcare services may turn out differently between countries, even though the overall aim in each country is the same: optimal outcomes for their population.

In this chapter we will first introduce complexity theory and how it can help to understand the dynamic processes that shape care services. Subsequently, we will describe the development of one specific maternity care service: fetal screening in three countries – Iceland, the Netherlands and the United Kingdom – and use complexity theory to reflect on this process.

Complexity theory: an introduction

In current healthcare, the linear focus of 'normal science' is unable to adequately account for the complex interactions that direct the provision of services. There is a turn towards complexity theory as a more appropriate framework for understanding system behaviour. Complexity theory was first developed as a way of understanding and taking into account discrepancies in physics (Plsek & Greenhalgh, 2001; Prigogine, 1997). It specifically marked a shift from classic linear science towards a more dynamic approach to science.

Over the last decennia complexity theory has been applied to many other scientific fields, to explain phenomena in biology, economics and social systems. There has been a growing interest in applying complexity theory in the healthcare context since 2001, when the *British Medical Journal* launched a series of articles on complexity in healthcare (Plsek & Greenhalgh, 2001; Wilson, Holt & Greenhalgh, 2001; Plsek & Wilson, 2001; Fraser & Greenhalgh, 2001). The argument is made that healthcare organisations can be viewed as complex adaptive systems (Committee on Quality Health Care in America, Institute of Medicine, 2001).

To understand the nature of complexity in healthcare systems, we used the taxonomy of complexity theory we have built and tested in a former study (Nieuwenhuijze *et al*, 2015). This taxonomy is grounded on complexity theory components from 31 publications identified in a systematic review of the literature on complexity theory and healthcare. The final taxonomy included and defined 11 components that characterise complex adaptive systems. These components are presented below: interconnection, open boundaries, initial conditions, simple rules, self-organisation, feedback loops, emergence, non-linearity, unpredictability, attractors, and co-evolution (Nieuwenhuijze *et al*, 2015).

Taxonomy

The behaviour of a complex system emerges from one of its fundamental characteristics: it includes a dynamic range of agents (e.g. people) who are *interconnected* and interact through (local) interdependent relationships and free flow of information. Each of the agents is connected to various other systems through *open boundaries*. Systems cannot be screened off from their environment. People, information, and ideas move across the various systems. Individual agents are part of several systems at the same time, and membership of systems changes over time. Interconnection also facilitates *feedback loops* in which the positive and/or negative effects of a particular action or change are fed back to the people in the system. The feedback affects the way people will behave in the future, also in the connection with one another.

However, complex systems also have a history. This history constitutes the *initial conditions* that co-create the system's present behaviour and influence whether changes occur.

The interconnectivity between people stimulates *self-organisation* as a spontaneous process in which people mutually adapt their behaviour to cope with changing internal and external demands and thereby change the system. This behaviour is guided by *simple rules* as internalised principles or values driving a common direction of travel among people in a complex system. These rules are general enough to provide space for shared action and innovative change.

A complex system emerges over time, adapting flexibly in response to internal and external challenges. This results in new patterns of behaviour, in which the whole is greater than the sum of the parts. *Emergence* is enhanced by diversity in the interconnection. The changes that occur in complex systems are *non-linear*. When changes happen, the cause-effect relationships are usually not self-evident or linear. Small changes can have large, non-proportional effects on the whole system (and vice versa). The behaviour of any complex system is *unpredictable*. How exactly the systems will evolve and will be operating at any given time cannot be predicted in detail. Because of random disturbances, non-linearity of changes and emergent behaviour open to feedback, accurate detailed planning is impossible.

The system eventually settles after a period of turbulence. Over time, new structures and patterns emerge without hierarchical direction. The system will be operating within certain parameters ('phase space'). A *strange attractor* is the emerged new set of behaviours of the system, within a 'phase space'.

A complex system co-evolves with its environment, because it is embedded in other systems. *Co-evolution* is a process of mutual transformation, initiated by continuous change in the environment which requires new responses and approaches. The evolution of each of these complex systems influences and is influenced by the evolution of other systems.

The components are strongly connected. The links can be distinguished at three levels: (1) components at the system level: which trigger (2) a process characterised by certain components: leading to (3) an outcome which has a number of characteristic components (Figure 1).

Figure 1. Relationship scheme of the taxonomy of complex systems

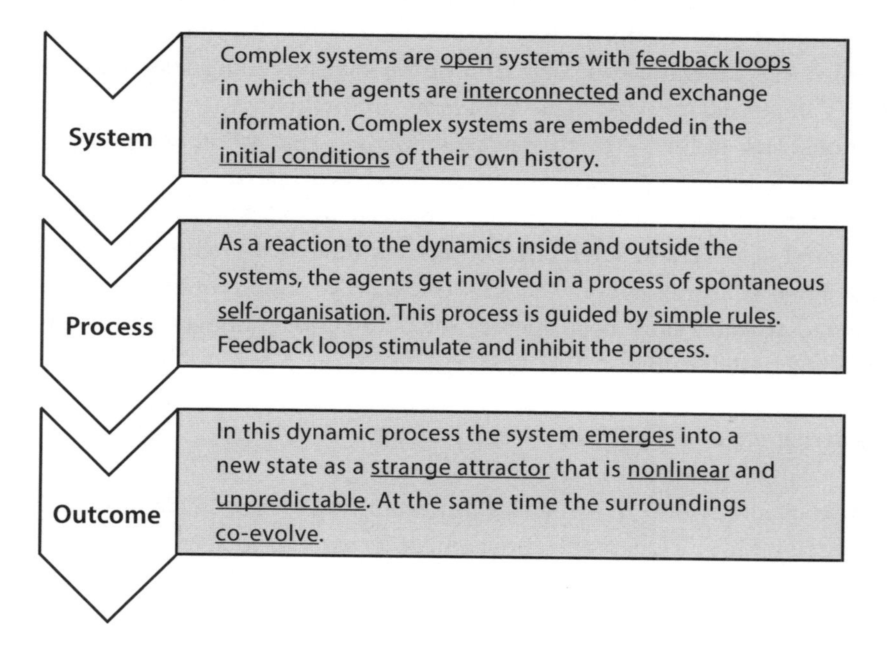

We will use these concepts from complexity theory to generate practical insights into the development of antenatal screening – in particular, fetal screening – and to enable a better understanding of differences in services among countries.

Development of fetal screening in Iceland, the Netherlands and the United Kingdom

In general, screening is a systematic attempt to select those who are at high risk of a specific disease from among apparently healthy individuals (Cuckle, 2004). As such the aim of screening is prevention. Decisions about care are based on information so timely interventions can be provided (Hornnes, 2010). Screening can be performed with a number of methods although all screening programmes have three components: test, disease and preventive action (Cuckle, 2004). An underlying impetus for the increasing emphasis on screening is the risk discourse, which is an integral part of today's healthcare. Some have argued that this emphasis has gone too far resulting in a 'risk epidemic' or 'risk society' which is the subject of much controversy (Beck-Gernsheim, 2002; Solbekken, 1995). At the core of this debate are the different interpretations of available evidence and uncertainty about the effectiveness of some screening procedures.

Antenatal screening can refer to a number of screening tests used to identify maternal and/or fetal problems in pregnancy (e.g. anaemia, infections, lack of fetal growth). In the following description we limit our discussion to fetal screening (FS), specifically referring to the combined test (nuchal translucency measuring and biochemical markers) and the 20-week ultrasound scan. These screening procedures have developed differently in the three countries where the 20-week scan is widely offered but the combined test has only been incorporated in some countries or regions during the past decades.

Fetal screening and diagnosis – historical path

The use of ultrasound in obstetrics in the mid-1950s can be defined as a starting point for FS where the initial aim of its use was to detect anomalies and measure gestational age. Donald *et al* were the first to introduce diagnostic ultrasound to obstetrics and gynaecology in the late fifties (Donald, Macvicar & Brown, 1958) and in the following years several new methods and parameters for examining the fetus and measuring the length of pregnancy using ultrasound were introduced (Campbell & Wilkin, 1975; Robinson & Shaw-Dunn, 1973). Following the discovery by the French cytogeneticist Jerome LeJeune in 1959 that Down's syndrome is due to an extra chromosome number 21, amniocentesis was developed and, in 1968, the first prenatal diagnosis of Down's syndrome by amniocentesis was reported in the UK (Valenti, Schutta & Kehaty, 1968). Increased flexibility in abortion policy at that time in a number of countries, such as the US, the UK and Canada, encouraged the development of FS procedures such as amniocentesis (Louhiala, 2004). As medical and genetic technology evolved during the last part of the 20th century and the beginning of the 21st, new procedures in FS emerged. The development of nuchal translucency screening (NT) was described as a method where the space between the skin and the cervical spine of the fetus is measured in a sagittal view. An increased NT is associated with a raised risk of trisomy 21 as well as other chromosomal abnormalities, major heart defects and a wide range of skeletal dysplasia and genetic syndromes (Nicolaides, Heath & Liao, 2000; Spencer, 2000). Most parents experience FS as positive (Gottfredsdottir, Sandall & Björnsdottir, 2009; Jaques, Sheffield & Halliday, 2005; Muller *et al*, 2006). A handful of studies show that decisions on screening are not based on adequate knowledge although that is seen as the key component of informed choice (Jaques, Sheffield & Halliday, 2005; Michie, Dormandy & Marteau, 2005). However, women with higher education and income status seem to have better knowledge about screening which is reflected in the finding that women with lower income and educational levels are more likely to make an uninformed choice (Jaques, Sheffield & Halliday 2005; Gourounti & Sandall, 2008).

With a continuing development in screening methods, a procedure with cell-free fetal DNA/RNA in maternal plasma being present as early as four weeks of gestation has been introduced as non-invasive prenatal testing (NIPT) (Lewis *et al*, 2014). In practice, it can now identify pregnancies with Down's, Edwards' and Patau's syndrome from ten weeks with a low false positive rate (Chiu *et al*, 2011). It is likely that it will be possible to detect other anomalies in future. Women are generally positive about this method. The high level of accuracy and the reduced number of pregnant women who will have invasive testing are appealing to healthcare providers. However, a number of concerns have been raised related to the ease and frequency of these blood tests (Hall, Bostanci & John, 2009). First, as early NIPT is a safe and easy method; informed choice may become more difficult. Consequently both testing and selective abortion will become 'normalised'. Second, NIPT for a broad range of abnormalities might induce a trend towards accepting testing for minor abnormalities and non-medical traits. This will generate a large amount of information and inevitably include findings that will be difficult to interpret and explain (De Jong *et al*, 2010). For professionals who are not specialised in the area of genetics it will be a challenge to provide adequate and understandable counselling both pre- and post-screening.

These advancements in science will sooner or later present the question of where we draw the line when it becomes possible to detect less serious anomalies and non-medical traits.

The Icelandic story

The development of maternity care in Iceland followed the main trends seen in Europe and the US, and today the organisation of maternity care is similar to many European countries where women seek antenatal care within healthcare centres and the majority give birth in hospitals. Iceland shares the Nordic identity of a welfare state meaning that antenatal care is free of charge, except if a woman chooses to go to a private obstetrician. The health policy in the country is characterised by strong state involvement, where the majority of healthcare institutions and community centres are governmentally run. However, some services are privately run although costs are (partly) covered by national health insurance. Private practice provided by obstetricians exists for reproductive health, but is more or less limited to the initial pregnancy assessment. Most parents use the services provided at the community centres once pregnancy has been established. Other services, such as delivery and postpartum care, are free but antenatal classes are paid for by prospective parents. The midwife is the main caregiver in the 'normal' process of pregnancy and childbirth, and all Icelandic midwives are licensed to practise independently (Regulation on Health Care Centres, 2014).

There were 4450 births in Iceland in 2012, and the home birth rate was 2.2%, the highest in the Scandinavian countries (Bjarnadottir *et al*, 2013). During that year caesarean sections were 15.4% and instrumental deliveries 8.6%. Childbearing is highly valued in the country and this is reflected in the fact that 39% of childbearing women are having their first child, compared to 50-53% in Italy, Spain and the UK (European Perinatal Health Report, 2012). In 2012, Icelandic women gave birth to 2.04 children and at the same time maternal age at delivery was 35 years or more for 18.9% of childbearing women in Iceland and is still increasing (Bjarnadottir *et al*, 2013).

Fetal screening in Iceland – past and present

Due to a relatively small population, the development of FS in Iceland provides a good opportunity to explore how the interaction between healthcare policy, clinical professionals and prospective parents has evolved. The use of ultrasound at 20 weeks for all women was initiated at the Women's Clinic at Landspitali University Hospital in 1975, and in 1978 amniocentesis became available for women aged 35 and over. Today, eight units in the country offer a 19-20-week scan, free of charge. In 1999, NT screening was introduced as a new screening method for women over 35 years of age in order to reduce the use of amniocentesis but, by 2005, the screening had become established practice in the country with about 84.5% of prospective mothers opting for it in the capital area, i.e., where there is easy access (Gottfredsdottir, Sandall & Björnsdottir, 2009). Although several meetings and study days took place during the first years when the screening was being implemented no official working group was formed with the specific role to evaluate and recommend about follow up. It was not until 2006 that official recommendations on the screening were issued by the Director of Health (Directorate of Health, 2006), and clinical guidelines were developed in 2008. There was, however, a considerable debate among the various professionals concerning the matter, especially regarding information and counselling for women/parents, which some professionals saw as a prerequisite to implementation. In Iceland the equity principle has been the driving force as emphasised in 'the Nordic healthcare model', although a recent analysis of the Nordic healthcare systems shows that the reality is considerably more complex as the shift of political power to centre-right wing has been associated with changing policies about patients' rights and increased consumer freedom to choose (Magnussen, Vrangbæk & Saltman, 2009). Screening uptake in the country varies by place of residence, as was shown in a study based on data from 2009 and 2010. In the capital area 87% of women had the test or were going to accept it during that time, 70% of women living in the north of Iceland, 62% of women in the east part, but only 29% of women from an area in the west of Iceland (Kormaksdottir, 2013). One can speculate if this is related to access or a difference in the pathway of care and information. A small qualitative study conducted in the capital area showed that the decision to decline is largely determined by what prospective parents bring with them to the pregnancy, i.e., their personal philosophy of Down's syndrome and the high value they place on maintaining the complexity of life (Gottfredsdottir, Sandall & Björnsdottir, 2009). Prospective parents pay for the NT screening in Iceland (€69.00) which was meant to underline that the offer of screening was optional. Informed choice in this context is emphasised in the national clinical guidelines for antenatal care. However, although studied to a limited degree, only 57% of prospective mothers believe they have sufficient knowledge about NT screening (Stefansdottir *et al*, 2010), and women who accept screening are likely to view the offer as a part of antenatal care (Gottfredsdottir, Sandall & Björnsdottir, 2009)

When the screening was implemented in the country no official guidelines or policy existed around its use. Iceland is a small country and the knowledge about this new test quickly spread among women. The test developed in a short time from a test for a limited group (women over 35) to a 'screening for all policy'. Initially, before guidelines came into place, FS was mainly promoted by staff at the specialised clinic where the test was offered and which had a strong connection with departments of fetal medicine in the UK where the staff at the department sought their training. Concerns about FS have been brought up on a regular basis following news concerning the abortion rate of fetuses with DS both by parents and organisations of DS children, and a critical debate regarding the routine use of NT screening took place. However, an analysis of the discourse in the Icelandic media around the implementation of FS showed that the societal response was fairly muted and it did not change the development of FS in Iceland. The overall pattern is that, for the last decades, the majority of women in Iceland have accepted the FS that is offered.

Fetal screening in the future

The development in non-invasive prenatal testing (NIPT) has evoked very little debate among the public or professionals about this new procedure. However, some change is already in the air as women search for information on the internet during pregnancy and therefore are aware of new possibilities in this context. A study conducted in the UK showed that women and health professionals have different values towards test accuracy and safety when it comes to making a decision about NIPT (Hill *et al*, 2012). That supports the need to explore this further in countries where this test could be implemented in the coming years.

A complexity reflection on the development of fetal screening in Iceland

Looking back on the development of FS in Iceland one can say that it was initiated by the staff in the Department of Fetal Diagnosis in one specific hospital (Landspitali University Hospital) who had strong connections with health professionals in the UK (*self-organisation, interconnectivity*). Additionally, women wanted to have the same choice as offered in other countries (*open boundaries*). Absence of guidelines gave professionals the space to self-determine how to offer FS to women (*self-organisation*). Offering it to all women was rooted in the equity principle (*simple rules*) which has been the main emphasis in healthcare in Iceland (*initial conditions*) for decades. In the context of FS it has been interpreted as a 'screening for all policy'. Payment for the NT screening underlines the fact that the offer of screening is optional (*simple rules*). Although concerns have been raised regarding the development of FS, the pattern that the majority of women accept what is offered in FS has been established in Iceland *(strange attractor)*. Variations in the uptake of FS in Iceland show that the delivery of care affects the uptake of screening *(unpredictability)*.

Recently, as women have become aware of new tests through the internet (*open boundaries*) it seems logical that the offer of the recent NIPT will be supported both on the macro and micro level in Iceland.

The Dutch story

In 2012, there were 173,099 births in the Netherlands including 16.3% caesarean sections and 9.2% instrumental deliveries. The fertility rate among women was 1.7 children per woman in 2012. At birth, 0.1% of the women were younger than 18 and 20.5% were 35 years or more. In total, 26% of the women were of non-Dutch origin (Utrecht: Stichting Perinatale Registratie Nederland, 2013).

Dutch maternity care is based on the principle that pregnancy and childbirth are fundamentally physiological processes (College voor Zorgverzekeringen, 2003). The care system includes independent midwives in the community providing care to healthy women with uncomplicated pregnancies and births, and obstetricians responsible for the care of high-risk women in the hospital setting. Both have been recognised as medical professionals by Dutch law since 1865 (Wet op de beroepen in de individuele gezondheidszorg, 1993), and each care provider is individually registered with a government agency (Cronie, Rijnders & Buitendijk, 2013).

Around 85% of all women in the Netherlands start their care in pregnancy with a midwife (Utrecht: Stichting Perinatale Registratie Nederland, 2013). Healthy women with an uncomplicated pregnancy are free to follow their preference and give birth at home or in hospital under the supervision of their midwife. Midwives refer women to obstetric-led care when there is an increased risk of complications as defined by the 'List of Obstetric Indications', a national guideline, developed co-operatively by all the professions involved in maternity care (College voor Zorgverzekeringen, 2003). After referral, women may receive care from hospital midwives, obstetric residents, and obstetric nurses under the supervision of an obstetrician (Cronie, Rijnders & Buitendijk, 2013).

Basic health insurance is legally mandatory for all Dutch residents. Health insurance is offered by a number of commercial insurance companies, which are regulated by a government body. Financial compensation is available for low-income groups. The basic insurance covers all the costs of maternity care; there is no excess payment unless a healthy woman chooses a midwifery-led hospital birth. In that case, a woman makes a co-payment of approximately €300 for the additional costs of the hospital stay. Some insurance plans cover these costs. This underscores the physiological orientation towards birth.

Fetal screening in the Netherlands – past and present

In the Netherlands, tests for the detection of fetal anomalies became available in the 1970s. Initially, all women over 37 years of age, and from 1985 all women over 35 years, were offered the option of amniocentesis or chorionic villus sampling to detect Down's syndrome, Patau's and Edwards' syndrome and – in the case of amniocentesis – neural tube defects. Women with a personal or family history of listed congenital anomalies are offered testing regardless of their age. Health professionals (midwives, family physicians or obstetricians) who conduct the antenatal intake provide information and support women in their decision-making. The tests are performed in eight genetic centres in the Netherlands (Brief van de Minister van Volksgezondheid, 1996).

General use of ultrasound started in the second half of the 1970s. As the image quality improved, it was increasingly used for detection purposes in women with a higher risk of a fetus with structural anomalies, e.g. heart defects. Until the end of the 20th century, these specialised ultrasounds were mainly performed in the genetic centres. Ultrasounds were not offered systematically to all women for screening of congenital anomalies.

At the end of the 1980s, the idea of introducing FS at the population level was introduced, but was met with unease in the Netherlands. Maternity care professionals and patient organisations were divided concerning the screening test. This led to strong debates among health professionals and in the public domain, such as parliament and the media. Dialogue and seeking consensus on ethically sensitive areas is necessary as the Dutch public domain is characterised by Christian moral principles as well as social–democratic and liberal influences. Parliament plays an active role in initiating these discussions.

The government's position in the debates on FS gave cause for concern. Unintentionally, the impression was raised that the government wanted to use genetic services to improve public health and reduce the costs of healthcare through preventive abortion of fetuses with severe abnormalities. This evoked associations with eugenic population policies from the first half of the 20th century (Van El, Pieters & Cornel, 2012). In May 1988, the Minister of Health reassured the country that there was no need for concerns about the government's policy on prenatal testing and the position of disabled people in Dutch society. The birth of a disabled child would never be regarded as a case of failed prevention (Parliamentary documentation. Tweede Kamer der Staten-Generaal, 1987-1988b). The government explicitly stated that pressure from professionals or public opinion should not constrain the option of parents not taking a test (Parliamentary documentation. Tweede Kamer der Staten-Generaal, 1989-1990a). The Minister of Health decided against nationwide FS, based on considerations of technical, organisational and ethical grounds (Meijer *et al*, 2010; Parliamentary documentation. Tweede Kamer der Staten-Generaal, 1991-1992). The large number of false positive results with the triple test was seen as unsuitable for population screening. This would cause unnecessary anxiety among many pregnant women and increasing medicalisation of maternity care. Also the decentralised healthcare system made it hard to facilitate access to FS for all pregnant women. However, the most important barrier was abortion as the only 'treatment' option in many cases. Abortion as a treatment was considered controversial (Meijer *et al*, 2010). Population screening was only meant for early identification of *treatable* conditions (Wet op Bevolkingsonderzoek, 1996). In parliament, all parties from the left to right wing supported the government's decision not to implement nationwide screening (Parliamentary documentation. Tweede Kamer der Staten-Generaal, 1989-1990b).

Around the turn of the century, opinions about FS shifted. Treatment was no longer an absolute criterion; screening also became acceptable for other 'practical courses of action' (Health Council of the Netherlands, 2001). Additionally, population screening was no longer considered an instrument only for collective prevention, but also an instrument that enabled individuals to make decisions for personal reasons. The patient's right to self-determination gained more weight in the discussions on FS. The overall aim of FS became offering a well-informed choice to pregnant women, on which they could decide in accordance with their personal preferences. Adequate information and counselling were explicitly mentioned as conditions that guaranteed public acceptability of FS. The growing reliability of new non-invasive tests made access to FS for all pregnant women desirable from an equality of rights perspective.

Finally, in 2004, the government decided that FS should become available to all women. After decades of discussion and various reports from the Health Council (Health Council of the Netherlands, 2001; Health Council of the Netherlands, 1989; Health Council of the Netherlands, 2004), there was enough support among all the parties involved – professionals, the Health Council, patient organisations and the government – to establish FS on Down's syndrome as a nationwide programme. All women over 35 years of age are informed of the possibility of FS, but younger women receive information on FS only at their explicit request. This last restriction was criticised by professionals and evoked many questions in parliament (Kleiverda, 2004; van Huis, 2004; van der Putten, 2003; Parliamentary documentation. Tweede kamer der Staten General, 2003-2004). In January 2007, a national screening programme emerged: all women are now asked if they want to be informed about FS. This resulted in a stable situation with little debate in recent years. Well-informed choice is still greatly emphasised. Women are counselled by their healthcare professional if they want to receive information and, based on the information provided, the woman decides whether or not she wants to opt for screening. She is offered the first-trimester combined test for the detection of Down's syndrome and the fetal anomaly scan at 18-22 weeks of gestation for the detection of structural anomalies (RIVM website, 2014). Women over 35 years of age are offered a choice between the combined test and invasive diagnostic testing.

FS is part of insured care for women over 35 years of age. Younger women pay for the combined test which costs approximately €150. However, from 1st January 2015 all women, regardless of age, will have to pay for the combined test. The anomaly scan is free of charge for all women. Any follow up based on the test results is also paid for by the insurance. Well-informed decision-making and counselling have been an important part of FS. This is done at the start of antenatal care by the maternity care providers, who are all specifically trained for this. Careful, non-directive information plays an important part in the decision-making process, which respects the right of not knowing, and gives pregnant women enough time for consideration. The information needs to enhance well-considered and voluntary choices.

Since the availability of the combined test, the uptake has been around 23-32%, whereas the uptake of the fetal anomaly scan has been between 90-95% (Engels, 2014; Gitsels *et al*, 2014a; Bakker *et al*, 2012). The effect on the uptake of prenatal diagnostic testing for women over 36 years of age has been minimal, with only a 10% decrease being seen (Engels, 2014).

The participation rate for the combined test is low in the Netherlands, but the national screening programme is not directed at achieving high uptake rates. More important is whether the uptake rate is based on informed decision-making (Engels, 2014). Several studies have taken place in the Netherlands. Neither uptake rates nor the attitude towards FS of pregnant women were significantly predicted by counsellors' attitudes towards FS (van den Berg *et al*, 2007). The large majority of women reported that they made the decision autonomously (Bakker *et al*, 2012). High levels of informed decision-making were demonstrated and information provision on the combined test was of good quality. However, one study reported that women often did not have adequate knowledge on the combined test (Schoonen *et al*, 2012).

Great variance in uptake is seen between regions and practices. The way health professionals present the tests might explain the difference, but also ethnic or religious differences in the populations (Gitsels *et al*, 2014a; Bakker *et al*, 2012). The participation rate for the combined test was lower in specified non-western ethnic minorities (Fransen *et al*, 2010) although, another study showed that non-western women with limited provision of Dutch were more likely to take the combined test (Gitsels *et al*, 2014a). There are indications that religion (Islam, Protestantism) plays a role in declining the combined test (Gitsels *et al*, 2014a; Gitsels *et al*, 2014b).

For the majority of women, the reason for declining the combined test was their attitude towards Down's syndrome – not finding it a reason to terminate pregnancy – and a negative attitude towards abortion (Bakker *et al*, 2012).

Fetal screening in the future

So far, little public debate has taken place around the ethical issues of NIPT in the Netherlands. NIPT is currently only available through a nationwide study, and only women with a higher risk for Down's syndrome are eligible. Recently, however, the test has been offered commercially in neighbouring countries, advertising it on the internet. Women have turned to laboratories in Belgium or Germany for access to the test, where they will have to pay approximately €800-1000.

A complexity reflection on the development of fetal screening in the Netherlands

Development of FS in the Netherlands was the result of interaction between different agents, such as patients' organisations, professional organisations, the media, the Health Council, and the Dutch parliament and government (*interconnectivity*). Steps in the implementation were adjusted based on the reactions of the public and professionals (*feedback loops*). The character of the Dutch public domain, as well as technical and organisational conditions, influenced the implementation process (*initial conditions*). Ethical principles, such as well-informed decision-making and safeguarding the right not to take the test (*simple rules*), had a great impact. Uptake of FS has been unexpectedly low so far, considering the high amount of debate it has evoked over the last decades (*non-linearity, unpredictability*).

Initially, the government was leading the way in which FS was offered. In 2007 a national programme emerged and a relatively stable situation was achieved (*emergence, strange attractor*). However, free flow of information through social media, open access to healthcare in other countries (*open boundaries*), and the recent commercial offering of new tests (NIPT) (*co-evolution*) has let to women seeking this new test in other countries (*self-organisation*). The likely possibilities of this new test make it hard to foretell what FS will look like in the future (*unpredictability*).

The UK story

Maternity care in the UK (comprising of England, Scotland, Wales and Northern Ireland, all of which have slightly different systems) is largely provided by the National Health Service (NHS), which is free at the point of delivery and paid for from general taxation. There are approximately 700,000 births each year in England (Care Quality Commission, 2013). For the majority of women, especially prima gravidas, the first point of contact is their general practitioner (GP), with 63% seeing their GP and 32% seeing a midwife as the first point of contact with a healthcare practitioner. Most women see a midwife for antenatal check-ups (98%) and 42% also see a consultant. Booking for maternity services is usually before the 12th week: 53% of women see a healthcare professional before they are six weeks pregnant, 44% between 7-12 weeks, and 4% after 13 weeks (Care Quality Commission, 2013). Most women give birth in hospitals; 2.3% of women gave birth at home in England and Wales in 2013 (ONS, 2014). The 30-34 age group had the highest number of deliveries (29.7% of deliveries). Caesarean section rates are at 25.5% putting England in the higher level of caesarean rates in Europe (HES, 2013).

Currently screening guidelines in the UK state that women should be routinely offered an ultrasound for fetal abnormality at 18-20 weeks, and the combined test for Down's should be offered between 11 and 13 weeks. For women who book later, or when it is not possible to measure the nuchal translucency, the triple or quadruple test should be offered between 15 and 20 weeks (NICE, 2010). In the guidance it is made clear that, 'women should be given information about the purpose and implications of the anomaly scan to enable them to make an informed choice as to whether or not to have the scan' (NICE, 2010).

Fetal screening in the UK – past and present

With developments in ultrasound technology the use of ultrasound in obstetric practice began to increase from the late 1950s onwards. By 1966 it was reported that 28% of obstetric patients in Donald's Glasgow centre were receiving ultrasound (Oakley, 1986). Stuart Campbell, one of Donald's team, brought the technology to England in 1968 (Campbell, 2010). By the early 1970s about half of the women in his hospital had an ultrasound, and by 1978 most of the women did. By the late 1970s obstetric ultrasound had become a relatively common procedure for monitoring fetal growth and maturity. Ultrasound technology enabled the monitoring of the fetus and the doctor could 'see' the baby. The mother was no longer the custodian of fetal experience; this could now be observed directly. With this direct access to the baby, obstetrics became more concerned with the baby rather than maternal health, as Donald noted in his textbook, *Practical Obstetric Problems*: 'In place of maternal mortality, perinatal mortality has now become the yardstick by which we review our work. This is at least a sound beginning which acknowledges our custodianship of the baby's future' (Donald, 1964). Editions of the Myles midwifery textbook published in the early 1970s included a new section on perinatal health reflecting this new emphasis on the fetus (Myles, 1971).

Since its inception, the use of ultrasound in pregnancy has moved from being a diagnostic test for pregnancies at risk to a general screening tool for all pregnancies – all pregnancies are now subject to surveillance in this way. This is part of the technological impetus that once something is introduced for one category of woman (i.e., those at risk) it gains momentum and becomes applied to other areas. Further, women like the ability to 'see' their baby, as evidenced by the increasing availability of 4D scans that are offered privately and produce a 'better' picture of the baby. The introduction of general screening was a gradual process and ultrasound did not become routine in practice till the late 1990s. In the late 1980s such screening was still not routine and only offered to women in recognised risk groups (Luck, 1992). By the early 2000s an ultrasound at 18-20 weeks was being recommended for all women (National Collaborating Centre for Women's Health, 2003).

There was consumer opposition to the increased use of screening and monitoring of otherwise normal pregnancies. One of the main issues was that the use of ultrasound in pregnancy had not been evaluated and there were concerns that it could present a risk to the fetus. The Association for Improvements in the Maternity Services (AIMS) (AIMS, 1995) wrote to the Minister of Health in 1982 to express concerns over this (Beech, 2013).

> *It is a disgrace that for the last 35 years women have been taking part in the largest unevaluated medical experiment of all time. They are being used as guinea pigs in the medical profession's enthusiasm to find out as much as possible about the workings of the uterus and the developing fetus. Despite years of consumer pressure little is being done to inform women properly and address growing informed lay concerns.*
> (AIMS, 1995)

Other concerns were that women were not informed that the purpose of the scans was to detect abnormalities. Instead they were told that they were going to 'see' their baby and were often unprepared for the possibility of bad news. As with many issues in maternity care, the public voice was not of one opinion on the issues raised by this new technology. Disability groups questioned the premise of such screening. There were campaigns by AIMS and the National Childbirth Trust (NCT) against the use of technology but, as Jean Robinson from AIMS noted, campaigning against ultrasound was not easy as it was popular with women in the way other interventions such as induction were not (McIntosh, 2013). Current public concerns over screening in pregnancy are now about lack of access to the newest techniques rather than concerns over too much screening (*The Guardian*, 2009). Screening provision is not uniform across the UK, with some areas getting the newer tests before others, due to the way the NHS is organised (with geographical areas having their own commissioning groups who commission different ranges of services and may delay implementing new techniques due to funding constraints). There are also criticisms that there is a 'postcode' lottery, and that the tests you get depend on where you live rather than clinical need. Not all parts of the UK have implemented all of the National Institute for Health and Care Excellence's (NICE) screening recommendations. Often new developments might be available at a teaching hospital in a big city and not in smaller regional hospitals.

There is a lack of national data on the prevalence of ultrasounds and timings in the UK. The Maternity Services Data Set began in 2014 and is collecting data on the take up of dating scans, fetal anomaly scans and antenatal screening tests. A study in the early 2000s found that the mean number of ultrasounds per woman was 2.6 with 96% of women having at least one scan (Whynes, 2002). In June 2014 the UK National Screening Committee recommended that screening for trisomy 13 and 18 be screened for earlier in the first trimester rather than the current practice where it is screened for at the mid-point anomaly scan (UK National Screening Committee, 2014). Again, as this is a recent recommendation, there will be a time lag before it is implemented.

The combined test was introduced in the NHS around 1999. In 2008, the updated antenatal care NICE guidelines recommended that all women should be offered the combined test. However, it is still not widely available and roll out has been slow, for example, the NHS Lothian region in Scotland introduced the test in 2011 but it is not yet available on the NHS in Wales. In a national survey in 2010, 76% of women reported being screened by a blood test, nuchal fold or both, and 22% reported not wishing to have the tests. 'Most women felt they had a choice about the screening for Down's syndrome (93%) and that the reasons for screening had been clearly explained (93%), with no differences between women who had previously given birth and those who had not' (National Perinatal Epidemiology Unit, 2010). The vast majority, 90%, had a dating scan, 98.5% reported having a 20-week anomaly scan, and 85% reported having had a scan by 13 weeks or earlier (National Perinatal Epidemiology Unit, 2010).

Fetal screening in the future

The NIPT is only just trialled and is not generally available in the NHS, although it is available privately in the UK.

A complexity reflection on the development of fetal screening in the UK

The introduction of fetal screening in the UK started when doctors became interested in ultrasound techniques, and it steadily grew to become routine practice in many places *(self-organisation)*. Professionals getting connected at conferences *(interconnectivity)* and the free flow of information through specific journals like *Prenatal Diagnosis (open boundaries)* stimulated this development. There was some questioning of this uncontrolled, routine introduction of ultrasound by consumer organisations such as AIMS and the NCT, and disability groups questioned the premise of such screening *(self-organisation)*. Based on these concerns (*feedback loops),* the current guidelines emphasise that information must be given about the purpose and implications of FS to enable a well informed choice (*simple rules).* The basic premise of FS screening has now reached a stable situation where it is widely accepted by professionals and women *(strange attractor)*. The main tenor that now emerges emphasises the lack of access to 'new' technology in all regions *(emergence)*. Simultaneously, tests that are not available locally on the NHS can be purchased privately as well as 4D scans (*co-evolution).*

Overall reflection

In this chapter, we looked at the development of FS from a complexity theory perspective. Complexity theory can help us to understand what drives developments in modern, complex societies. The theory recognises that we must think outside linear models to understand more about the behaviour of healthcare systems, accept unpredictability, and respond flexibly to emerging patterns and opportunities (Plsek & Greenhalgh, 2001). This is illustrated by our example on the development of FS. It clearly shows that the introduction of new techniques in FS over the past decades has not been a linear process, i.e., the introduction of the ultrasound. Oakley gives a number of reflections on the introduction of ultrasound techniques for monitoring pregnancies (Oakley, 1986). Ultrasound entered in maternity care but it was actually developed for use in other areas of medicine. It quickly became part of routine practice, well before it had been evaluated and there had been any studies to determine its benefits and possible risk (the first RCT was in 1980). As obstetric ultrasound became a new part of practice, a professional structure of accreditation and professionalisation developed, such as the founding of the journal *Prenatal Diagnosis* in 1981.

This contributed to the creation of a new obstetric speciality and that again expanded its use.

We also found that FS has developed differently over time in Iceland, the Netherlands and the UK. In the Netherlands especially this has been a complex process with sensitive debates and a meandering evolution. In Iceland and the UK the implementation seems to have occurred in a more linear way with new tests being developed by medical professionals and subsequently offered to women. However, the Icelandic and British stories also show irregularities that do not fit into a linear idea, such as the regional differences in screening uptake of FS or the access to new tests. We found that nearly all the components from the taxonomy on complexity theory were present in our example.

Interconnectivity and *open boundaries* shaped the development of FS in all three countries. Free flow of information made both women and professionals aware of new possibilities and triggered their wish to have them available. In the UK and Iceland, it was the strong interconnection between the health professionals in these countries that influenced how FS developed. It was the medical staff that *self-organised* the introduction of FS in these countries. In the Netherlands, many different agents were involved in the discussions that influenced the timeframe and the steps in which FS was implemented. Initially, *self-organisation* around FS was limited in the Netherlands. The government claimed a determining role in the implementation process from the very start with specific laws and regulations. Their aim was to safeguard women's right to decline the use of FS and accept the chance of having a disabled child. Currently, the *open boundaries* in Europe and the internet have initiated new dimensions to self-organisation with Dutch women seeking access to the NIPT test abroad.

Initial conditions, are important as they affected the development of FS on a macro level in each country and, as such, shed light on the differences in how the process evolved. Pre-existing organisational situations or well established ideas on equity influenced the implementation process. *Feedback loops* helped to further shape the way FS is offered, with specific groups emphasising the importance of well informed choice and pushing towards accessibility of FS for all women.

The implementation process in all three countries was accompanied by *simple rules*. All claimed space for the notions that FS is optional and that women need to make a well informed choice. Changing policies about patients' rights and increased consumer freedom to choose played an important part in the process and how the availability of FS was finally shaped.

All countries have, after more or less turbulence, had a stable situation over the past years *(strange attractor)*. In theory, FS is now available for all women. However, there are still *non-linear* differences in uptake and accessibility of FS between and within these countries. It will be *hard to predict*, with new tests such as the NIPT coming up, what FS screening will look like in five years' time and whether it will evoke ethical discussions as it becomes easily accessible and available for minor abnormalities and non-medical traits.

Conclusion

Complexity theory helps us to understand what aspects played a role in the development of FS and make it clear that it was not a straightforward process but one that included many irregularities. *Interconnectivity, open boundaries* and *self-organisation* seem to have had an especially strong influence on the implementation process of FS. The complex behaviour of human beings and systems is something that is unescapably there and challenges us to work with it in an adaptable and flexible way.

References

AIMS (1995). *Ultrasound – the mythology of a safe and painless technology*. Available from: www.aims.org.uk/OccasionalPapers/ultrasoundTheMyth.pdf

Bakker M, Birnie E, Pajkrt E *et al* (2012). Low uptake of the combined test in the Netherlands – which factors contribute? *Prenat Diagn* 32: 1305-1312.

Beech B (2013). Ultrasound: prematurity and potential risks. *Midwifery Today* 105: 26-28. Available from: www.midwiferytoday.com/articles/ultrasound_risks.asp

Beck-Gernsheim E (2002). Health and responsibility: from social change to technological change and vice versa. In: Adam B, Beck U & Van Loon J (eds). *The Risk Society and Beyond*. London: Sage

Publications, pp122-135.

Bjarnadóttir RI, Garðarsdóttir G, Smárason, AK & Pálsson GI (eds) (2013). *Skýrsla frá fæðingaskráningunni fyrir árið 2012* [The Icelandic birth registration – Report for 2012]. Landspítali-háskólasjúkrahús (LUH), Reykjavik. Available from: www.landspitali.is/library/Sameiginlegar-skrar/Gagnasafn/Rit-og-skyrslur/Faedingaskraningar/faedingarskraning_skyrsla_2013.pdf

Brief van de Minister van Volksgezondheid, Welzijn en Sport [Letter from the Ministry of Health]. *Aan de Voorzitter van de Tweede Kamer der Staten-Generaal [To the chair of the* House of Representatives of the Dutch Parliament]. Rijswijk, March 1996.

Campbell S (2010). Early sonographic prenatal diagnosis. *Prenat Diagn* 30: 613-615.

Campbell S & Wilkin D (1975). Ultrasonic measurement of fetal abdomen circumference in the estimation of fetal weight. *Br J Obstet Gynaecol* 82: 689-697.

Care Quality Commission (2013). *National findings from the 2013 survey of women's experiences of maternity care.*

Chiu RW, Akolekar R, Zheng YW *et al* (2011). Non-invasive prenatal assessment of trisomy 21 by multiplexed maternal plasma DNA sequencing: large scale validity study. *BMJ* 342: 7401.

Cilliers P (1998). *Complexity & Postmodernism.* London: Routledge.

College voor Zorgverzekeringen (2003). *Verloskundig Vademecum.* Apeldoorn: VDA-groep.

Committee on Quality Health Care in America, Institute of Medicine (2001). *Crossing the quality chasm: a new health system for the 21st century.* Washington: National Academic Press.

Cronie D, Rijnders M & Buitendijk S (2013). Diversity in the scope and practice of hospital-based midwives in the Netherlands. *J Midwifery Women's Health* 57: 469-475.

Cuckle H (2004). Principles of screening. *The Obstetrician & Gynaecologist* 6: 21-25.

De Jong, A, Dondorp W, Die-Smulders C, Frints S & Wert G (2010). Non-invasive prenatal testing: ethical issues explored. *Eur J Hum Genet* 18: 272-277.

Directorate of Health. *Tilmæli um fósturskimun á meðgöngu* (2006). [Request regarding nuchal translucency screening during pregnancy]. Dreifibréf nr. 9 [Bulletin no. 9 of the Directorate of Health]. Directorate Health, Reykjavík. Available from: www.landlaeknir.is/Pages/207

Donald I (1964). *Practical Obstetric Problems.* 3rd edn. London: Lloyd-Luke.

Donald I, Macvicar J & Brown TG (1958). Investigation of abdominal masses by pulsed ultrasound. *Lancet* 7: 1188-1195.

Engels M (2014). *Prenatal Down syndrome screening: screening policies revised.* Proefschrift. Vrije Universiteit, Amsterdam.

Euro-Peristat Project with SCPE and Eurocat (2012). European Perinatal Health Report. The health and care of pregnant women and babies in Europe 2010. Brussels: Euro-Peristat. Available from: www.europeristat.com

Fransen MP, Schoonen MH, Mackenbach JP et al (2010). Ethnic differences in participation in prenatal screening for Down syndrome: a register-based study. *Prenat Diagn* 10: 988-994.

Fraser SW & Greenhalgh T (2001). Coping with complexity: educating for capability. *BMJ* 323: 799-803.

Gitsels-van der Wal JT, Verhoeven PS, Manniën J et al (2014a). Factors affecting the uptake of prenatal screening tests for congenital anomalies; a multicenter prospective cohort study. *BMC Pregnancy Childbirth* 14: 264.

Gitsels-van der Wal JT, Manniën J, Ghaly MM et al (2014b). The role of religion in decision-making on antenatal screening of congenital anomalies: a qualitative study amongst Muslim Turkish origin immigrants. *Midwifery* 30: 297-302.

Gottfredsdottir H, Sandall J & Björnsdottir K (2009). This is just what you do when you are pregnant. A qualitative study of prospective parents in Iceland who accept nuchal translucency screening. *Midwifery* 25: 711-720.

Gourounti K & Sandall J (2008). Do pregnant women in Greece make informed choices about antenatal screening for Down's syndrome? A questionnaire survey. *Midwifery* 24: 153-162.

The Guardian (2009). *NHS failure on Down's screening kills healthy babies.* 16 May.

Hall A, Bostanci A & John S (2009). Ethical, legal and social issues arising from cell-free fetal DNA technologies. Appendix III to the report: Cell-free fetal nucleic acids for non-invasive prenatal diagnosis. Cambridge: PHG Foundation.

Health Council of the Netherlands (2001). Prenatale screening: Downsyndroom, neuralebuisdefecten, routine-echoscopie [Prenatal screening: Down syndrome, neural tube defects, routine ultrasonography]. Publication no. 2001/11. The Hague: Health Council of the Netherlands.

Health Council of the Netherlands (1989). Erfelijkheid: maatschappij en wetenschap [Genetics: society and science]. The Hague: Health Council of the Netherlands.

Health Council of the Netherlands (2004). Prenatal screening (2): Downsyndroom, neuraalbuisdefecten' [Down's syndrome, neural tube defects]. Publication no. 2004/06. The Hague: Health Council of the Netherlands.

Hospital Episode Statistics (HES) (2013). *NHS Maternity Statistics 2012-13.*

Hill M, Fisher J, Chitty LS & Morris G (2012). Women´s and health professionals' preferences for prenatal tests for Down syndrome: a discrete choice experiment to contrast noninvasive prenatal diagnosis with current invasive tests. *Genet Med* 14 (11): 905-913.

Hornnes P (2010). EBCOG and the Nordic countries. *Acta Obstet Gynecol* 89: 297-298.

Jaques AM, Sheffield LJ & Halliday JL (2005). Informed choice in women attending private clinics to undergo first-trimester screening for Down syndrome. *Prenat Diagn* 25: 656-664.

Kormaksdottir G (2013). Er mundur á þjónustu fyrir verðandi foreldra varðandi fósturskimanir eftir búsetu? [Is the delivery of care in the context of fetal screening affected by parents' residence?]. Unpublished master's thesis. University of Iceland, Reykjavik.

Kleiverda G (2004). Kennis om te kunnen kiezen. Informatie over prenatale screening valt buiten deWBO [Knowledge to be able to choose. Information on prenatal screening goes outside the WBO]. *Medisch Contact* 59: 508-511.

Lewis C, Hill M, Silcock C, Daley R & Chitty L (2014). Non-invasive prenatal testing for trisomy 21: a cross-sectional survey of service users' views and likely uptake. *BJOG* 121: 582-594.

Louhiala P (2004). *Preventing Intellectual Disability.* Cambridge: Cambridge University Press.

Luck C (1992). Value of routine ultrasound scanning at 19 weeks. *BMJ* 304: 1474-1478.

Magnussen J, Vrangbæk K & Saltman RB (2009). *Nordic Health Care Systems. Recent Reforms and Current Policy Challenges.* London: Open University Press.

McIntosh T (2013). *A Social History of Maternity and Childbirth.* London: Routledge.

Meijer S, Stemerding D, Hoppe R et al (2010). Prenatale screening: een (on)getemd maatschappelijk probleem? [Prenatal screening: a (not yet) fully tamed problem?] *TSG* 88: 454-460.

Michie S, Dormandy E & Marteau TM (2005). Informed choice: understanding knowledge in the context of screening uptake. *Patient Educ Couns* 55: 218-222.

Muller MA, Bleker OP, Bonsel GJ & Bilardo CM (2006). Women's opinions on the offer and use of nuchal translucency screening for Down syndrome. *Prenat Diagn* 26: 105-111.

Myles M (1971). *A Textbook for Midwives*, 7th edn. Edinburgh: E & F Livingston Ltd.

National Collaborating Centre for Women's health (NCCWH) (2003). *Antenatal care: routine care for the healthy pregnant women.* Available from: www.nice.org.uk/guidance/cg62/evidence/evidence-tables-from-the-2003-version-196748322

National Perinatal Epidemiology Unit (2010). *Delivered with care: a national survey of women's experiences of maternity care in 2010.* Available from: www.npeu.ox.ac.uk/downloads/files/reports/Maternity-Survey-Report-2010.pdf

NICE (2010). *Antenatal care for uncomplicated pregancies: guidance 62.* Available from: www.nice.org.uk/guidance/cg62

Nicolaides KH, Heath V & Liao AW (2000). The 11-14 week scan. *Bailliere's Best Prac Res Clin Obstet Gynaecol* 14: 581-594.

Nieuwenhuijze MJ, Downe S, Gottfredsdottir H *et al* (2015). Taxonomy for complexity theory in the context of maternity care. *Midwifery* 31(9): 834-843.

Oakley A (1986). The history of ultrasonography. *Birth* 13: 8-13.

Office for National Statistics (ONS) (2014). *Births in England & Wales by characteristics of birth 2, 2013.*

Parliamentary documentation. Tweede Kamer der Staten-Generaal (1987–1988b). Preventie aangeboren afwijkingen. Verslag van een mondeling overleg [Prevention of congenital anomalies. Report of the oral discussion]. TK 20345:3.

Parliamentary documentation. Tweede kamer der Staten Generaal (1989–1990a). Bevolkingsonderzoek neuraalbuisdefecten. Brief van de Staatssecretaris van Welzijn, Volksgezondheid en Cultuur [Population screening for neural tube defects. Letter from the State Secretary of Welfare, Health and Culture]. TK 21353:1.

Parliamentary documentation. Tweede kamer der Staten Generaal (1991–1992). TK 21353:3.

Parliamentary documentation. Tweede kamer der Staten Generaal (1989–1990b). Bevolkingsonderzoek neuraalbuisdefecten. Verslag van een mondeling overleg [Population screening for neural tube defects. Report of the oral discussion]. TK 21353:2.

Parliamentary documentation. Tweede kamer der Staten Generaal (2003-2004). TK 29323:4.

Plsek PE & Greenhalgh T (2001). Complexity science: the challenge of complexity in health care. *BMJ* 323: 625-628.

Plsek PE & Wilson T (2001). Complexity, leadership, and management in healthcare organisations. *BMJ* 323: 746-749.

Prigogine I (1997). *The End of Certainty.* New York: Free Press, pp1-7.

Regulation on Health Care Centres no. 787/2007. [Reglugerð um heilsugæslustöðvar nr. 787/2007]. Available from: www.heilbrigdisraduneyti.is/log-og-reglugerdir/reglugerdir/nr/787

Robinson HP & Shaw-Dunn J (1973). Fetal heart rates as determined by sonar in early pregnancy. *J Obstet Gynaecol Br Commonw* 80: 805-809.

RIVM website: www.rivm.nl/en/Topics/P/Perinatal_screening.

Schoonen M, Wildschut H, Essink-Bot ML *et al* (2012). The provision of information and informed decision-making on prenatal screening for Down syndrome: a questionnaire- and register-based survey in a non-selected population. *Patient Educ Couns* 87: 351-359.

Solbekken JA (1995). The risk epidemic in medical journals. *Soc Sci Med* 40: 291-305.

Spencer K (2000). Second-trimester prenatal screening for Down's syndrome and the relationship for maternal serum biochemical markers to pregnancy complications with adverse outcome. *Prenat Diagn* 20: 652-656.

Stefansdottir V, Skirton H, Jonasson K, Hardardottir H & Jonsson J (2010). Effects of knowledge, education, and experience on acceptance of first trimester screening for chromosomal anomalies. *Acta Obstet Gynecol Scand* 89: 931-938.

Stichting Perinatale Registratie Nederland (2013). *Perinatale zorg in Nederland 2012 [Perinatale care in the Netherlands 2012]*. Utrecht: Stichting Perinatale Registratie Nederland.

UK National Screening Committee (2014). *Early screening for serious abnormalities in pregnancy to help women. News Release*. Available from: www.screening.nhs.uk/meetings

Valenti C, Schutta EJ & Kehaty T (1968). Prenatal diagnosis of Down's syndrome. *Lancet* 2: 220.

Wet op de beroepen in de individuele gezondheidszorg 1993 [Act on professions in individual healthcare 1993]. Available from: http://wetten.overheid.nl/BWBR0006251/geldigheidsdatum_11-11-2014

Wet op Bevolkingsonderzoek 1996 [Population Screening Act 1992]. Available from: http://wetten.overheid.nl/BWBR0005699/geldigheidsdatum_11-11-2014

Van El CG, Pieters T & Cornel M (2012). Genetic screening and democracy: lessons from debating genetic screening criteria in the Netherlands. *J Community Genet* 3: 79-89.

Van Huis M (2004). De politiek en prenatale screening [Politics and prenatal screening]. *Tijdschrift voor Verloskundigen* 3: 11-112.

Van der Putten M (2003). NTOG-AGORA: prenatale screening in Nederland [NTOG-AGORA: prenatal screening in the Netherlands]. *Nederlands Tijdschrift voor Obstetrie en Gynaecologie* 116: 341-344.

Van den Berg M, Timmermans DRM, Kleinveld A *et al* (2007). Are counsellors' attitudes influencing pregnant women's attitudes and decisions about prenatal screening? *Prenat Diagn* 27: 518–524.

Whynes D (2002). Receipt of information and women's attitudes to ultrasound scanning during pregnancy. *Ultrasound Obstet Gynaecol* 19: 7-12.

Wilson T, Holt T & Greenhalgh T (2001). Complexity science: complexity and clinical care. *BMJ* 323: 685-688.

CHAPTER 3

Core outcomes in maternity care research

Valerie Smith, Cecily Begley, Mechthild M. Gross and Declan Devane

Introduction

When designing studies, and randomised trials in particular, it is important to select outcomes that reflect the topic under study, are important for key stakeholders, will adequately inform answering the research question and will aid in determining the effects of interventions. In doing this, waste in research can be reduced and the potential to capitalise on the efficiency of research to improve health can be enhanced. It has been recognised, however, that the choice of outcomes in studies on similar topics across different areas of research is varied and inconsistent, presenting a significant challenge for researchers who wish to synthesise the evidence from these studies (Williamson *et al,* 2012). This challenge is further compounded when researchers measure the same outcome in a variety of ways (Clarke, 2007). While there is nothing comparable in progress in childbirth research, an example is available from schizophrenia. In an evaluation of 2,000 trials assessing 600 interventions in people with schizophrenia (Thornley & Adams, 1998), 640 various rating scales were used for measuring mental health wellbeing. In a follow-up report of 10,000 trials assessing 1,940 interventions relevant to the treatment of people with schizophrenia, 2,194 different instruments were used to measure mental health wellbeing (Miyar & Adams, 2012). Of these 2,194 instruments, 1,142 were used only once. Further adding to this problem is selective reporting of outcomes in research reports, which can lead to outcome reporting bias (Dwan *et al,*

2008; Smyth *et al*, 2010; Williamson & Clarke, 2012). Outcome reporting bias refers to the selection of a subset of a study's originally measured outcomes for reporting in study publications, on the basis of the strength and direction of their results (Hutton & Williamson, 2000), with positive/significant results more often being reported (Dickersin *et al*, 1987). The effect of this is that the published results of a study can be misleading as they do not truly reflect the study's complete results. In addition, outcome reporting bias can distort evidence synthesis in systematic reviews and meta-analyses, which are increasingly being relied on for informing healthcare decisions, resulting in potentially misinformed or inappropriate clinical decisions being made. The extent of this type of bias was highlighted recently in a review of 2,562 trials included in 283 Cochrane Reviews (Kirkham *et al*, 2010). Outcome reporting bias was suspected in at least one trial in 35% of the examined reviews. A sensitivity analysis, to assess the impact of this suspected bias, was performed using 81 of the 283 reviews that had a single meta-analysis of the review primary outcome. This analysis demonstrated that 64% (52/81) of these reviews included at least one trial that had a high suspicion for outcome reporting bias, and the treatment effect estimate was reduced by 20% or more in 23% (19/81) of the reviews (Kirkham *et al*, 2010). This demonstrates that outcome reporting bias can present a considerable problem for healthcare practitioners, decision-makers, and others, who wish to use the findings of Cochrane Reviews, other reviews, or individual trials, when making decisions about healthcare practice, policy and provision.

One of the suggested ways to address the difficulties presented by outcome variation and outcome reporting bias in systematic reviews, and other studies, is to develop and apply agreed sets of outcomes, known as 'core outcome sets' (COS) (Clarke, 2007; Williamson *et al*, 2012; The COMET Initiative, 2014). The idea here is that a COS represents the minimum that should be measured and reported in all clinical trials, or other studies, on a specific condition, while recognising that outcome measures outside of the COS might also be important in the context of each individual study. Developing and using COS in this way would facilitate increased synthesis of data from a number of studies on a specific condition, allow for meaningful comparisons of treatments and their effects to be made, and facilitate and encourage a more complete reporting of outcomes in studies (Turk *et al*, 2003; Dworkin *et al*, 2008; Williamson *et al*, 2012).

The focus of this chapter is on core outcomes in maternity care research. The need for COS in studies in maternity care is explored. Completed COS projects and plans for future COS on maternity care topics are discussed.

Lastly, initiatives from researchers interested in COS development, in healthcare in general and specific to maternity care, and methods for developing COS are described.

The case for core outcomes in maternity care research

Hundreds of thousands, even millions, of maternity care research studies have been conducted to date. All across the world, women are giving birth every day. How we care for these women, and their babies, is influenced heavily by cultural norms or by organisational, structural and economic constraints. In other instances, inconsistent, conflicting or unsubstantiated research evidence can impact on optimum maternity care provision. Using COS has the potential to minimise variation in the outcomes measured in studies on particular maternity care topics or conditions leading to an increased ability of reviewers to bring data on important outcomes together in a systematic review. This, in turn, has the potential to enhance the efficacy of research in maternity care, where higher levels of evidence on complete data sets can be achieved. However, previous and more recent work has identified variation and inconsistency in, and over pre-specifying pre-data collection with subsequent under-reporting of, outcomes in maternity care research. In this section, we discuss some aspects of this research to highlight and emphasise the case for COS in maternity care research.

Between August 2012 and March 2013, as part of a work plan within the Core Outcome Measures in Effectiveness Trials (COMET) Initiative, a survey of outcomes in 788 newly published 2007 and 2011 Cochrane Reviews, from 50 Cochrane Review Groups, was performed (Smith *et al*, 2015). In these 788 reviews, 6,127 outcomes were pre-specified in the methods sections of the reviews, and of these, when reviews with 0 included studies in them were excluded (86 reviews, 764 outcomes), 3,367 outcomes were reported (63%). This indicates that a substantial number of pre-specified outcomes are not being reported in Cochrane Reviews in general. Considering the Cochrane Pregnancy and Childbirth Group reviews in isolation (51 reviews), 592 outcomes were pre-specified in the methods sections of the reviews, and 289 of these (49%) were reported in the results sections. Furthermore, of the 51% of outcomes that were not reported, no reason was found in the text of the review for 19% of cases, suggesting, perhaps, that outcome reporting bias may be a problem in some Pregnancy and Childbirth Cochrane Reviews. Furthermore, Pregnancy and Childbirth Cochrane Reviews pre-specified a significantly greater number of outcomes than other Cochrane Review Groups. The median number of outcomes pre-specified across the 788 reviews was seven outcomes. The median number of specified outcomes in the reviews in the Pregnancy and Childbirth Group was substantially higher at 17 outcomes. Arguably, this might be explained and justified by considering that important and separate information on two individuals, a mother and a baby, is central to research in pregnancy and childbirth. This, in turn, may necessitate the use of extended lists of outcomes so that the relevant data, to answer the research question, can be captured. Whether this actually accounts for this finding or not, the important issue here is that the survey identified the Pregnancy and Childbirth Group as one of five review groups that reported less than 50% of their specified outcomes and the fourth lowest group, comparative to all Cochrane Review Groups, with respect to the proportion of specified outcomes that were being reported (Figure 1).

Figure 1:

Proportion of specified outcomes reported in the Cochrane Pregnancy and Childbirth Group (represented by the black column) reviews relative to all other Cochrane Review Groups

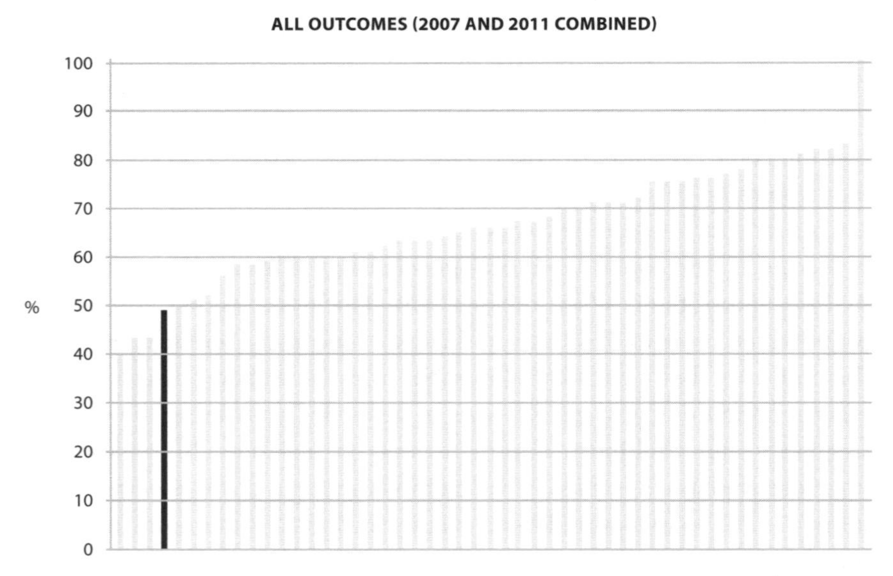

In addition, in a follow-up analysis of outcomes in newly published 2013 Cochrane Reviews (Wuytack *et al*, 2015), a negative correlation was found between the number of outcomes pre-specified in the methods sections of reviews and the proportion of these reported in the results sections ($r = -0.3$, $p<0.0001$), with reviews that pre-specified a larger number of outcomes reporting proportionately fewer outcomes in their results. This suggests that over-specifying with an associated under, or lack of, reporting of outcomes, selective reporting of outcomes, and/or considerable heterogeneity in outcomes measured in trials and in systematic reviews is, plausibly, causing a substantial problem for evidence synthesis in research in maternity care.

This latter suggestion of heterogeneity in outcomes in studies has been substantiated in a recent systematic review that investigated the differences in primary outcomes between randomised trials and systematic reviews in preterm birth prevention (Meher & Alfirevic, 2014). The review may go some way in explaining the findings from the survey of the Cochrane Pregnancy and Childbirth Group reviews, but, more importantly, it provides a clear example of where a lack of consensus and standardisation on choice of outcomes between trials and systematic reviews is impacting on evidence synthesis. The systematic review included a total of 170 studies and 33 systematic reviews on interventions for preventing preterm birth. Of the 170 trials, 103 (61%) pre-specified a primary outcome that was underpinned by a sample size calculation, and in these 103 trials, 72 different primary outcomes were reported. The most commonly reported outcome was preterm birth at <37 weeks gestation; reported in 12% (12/103) of trials; however, 58 of the 72 different outcomes (81%) were reported in one trial only. Of the 33 included systematic reviews or protocols, 82% (27/33) pre-specified more than one primary outcome, and 29 different primary outcomes were reported. Four of the nine most common primary outcomes in trials were never used as primary outcomes in reviews. These were latency of seven days (from exposure to intervention and birth), composite preterm birth and death, changes in contractions or cervical dilatation, and preterm birth <35 weeks. Similarly, 36% (4/11) of the most common primary outcomes reported in systematic reviews were not reported as primary outcomes in any of the trials. For example, *'death in baby'*, the most common primary outcome specified in the reviews, was reported as a primary outcome in 67% (22/33) of the reviews and in 1% (1/103) of the trials. Similarly, composite morbidity and mortality was reported in 30% (10/33) of the systematic reviews but in 5% (5/103) of the trials. Other examples of inconsistencies between trial and review outcomes include preterm birth <34 weeks (24% in reviews versus 3% in trials) and neonatal intensive care (NICU) admission for baby (9% in reviews versus 0% in trials).

Meher & Alfirevic's (2014) review reports on one condition in maternity care only and demonstrates a lack of consensus on what are the most important clinical outcomes related to preterm birth prevention. It is reasonable to assume, or at least to consider, that if one were to replicate this review using other conditions in maternity care, the results would possibly be similar in that we would likely find further evidence of heterogeneity in outcomes specified in trials and reviews on other specific conditions. Of visible interest in Meher & Alfirevic's (2014) review and in the survey of outcomes of Cochrane Pregnancy and Childbirth Group reviews (Smith *et al*, 2015) is the consistent mono-focus on adversity in the outcomes measured in studies in maternity care (Table 1 provides an illustrated example constructed using data from the survey of Cochrane Reviews).

Table 1:

Top 10 most frequently used outcomes in a sample of Cochrane Pregnancy and Childbirth reviews

2007 REVIEWS (N=19)		2011 REVIEWS (N=32)	
Outcome	No. of reviews using outcome (%)	Outcome	No. of reviews using outcome (%)
Neonatal/perinatal mortality	11 (58%)	Admission to NICU	15 (47%)
Adverse events/effects	10 (53%)	Maternal satisfaction	14 (44%)
Preterm birth <37 weeks	8 (42%)	Apgar <7 at 5mins	13 (41%)
Admission to NICU	6 (32%)	Perinatal mortality	13 (41%)
Postpartum haemorrhage	6 (32%)	Breastfeeding rate	11 (34%)
Severe neonatal morbidity	6 (32%)	Caesarean section	11 (34%)
Maternal mortality	5 (26%)	Instrumental birth	11 (34%)
Stillbirth	5 (26%)	Pain	10 (31%)
Maternal satisfaction	5 (26%)	Adverse events/effects	10 (31%)
Breastfeeding – initiation	4 (21%)	Infection	9 (28%)

Meeting the needs of low-risk mothers and their newborns: towards more health-focused outcomes in maternity

As part of our work within the COST Action (*IS0907 'Childbirth Cultures, Concerns, and Consequences: Creating a Dynamic EU Framework for Optimal Maternity Care'*) we explored this phenomenon through a systematic review of systematic reviews (Smith *et al*, 2014). The aim of the review was to identify the type and number of salutogenically focused reported outcomes reported in systematic reviews of intrapartum interventions. For the purpose of the review, we adopted a broad definition of the term 'salutogenesis' as it relates to optimum (and/or positive) maternal and neonatal health and wellbeing and defined a salutogenically focused outcome as *'an outcome reflecting positive health and wellbeing rather than illness or adverse event prevention or avoidance"* (Smith *et al*, 2014: 152).

Four hundred and thirty-six reviews published by the Cochrane Pregnancy and Childbirth Group were identified from Issue 9 (September 2011) of the Cochrane Database of Systematic Reviews. Of these reviews, through a process of independent screening and selection by pairs of reviewers and a complete-team consensus process, 102 were identified as intrapartum intervention-based reviews. Collectively, these 102 reviews reported 1767 outcomes. During the data extraction and analysis process, and through consensus meetings, 16 categories of salutogenically focused outcomes, involving 135 individual outcomes, were identified. Examples of these categories of outcomes include maternal satisfaction (reported 51 times), breastfeeding (initiation, duration or success) (reported 32 times), positive relationship with infant/bonding (reported six times), mobility during labour (reported three times) and comfort (reported twice). This compares unfavourably to 49 categories of non-salutogenically focused outcomes, involving 1,632 outcomes. Phrased alternatively, the results of the review found that the proportion of salutogenically focused outcomes compared to non-salutogenically focused outcomes in Cochrane Pregnancy and Childbirth Group reviews was 8% versus 92%. Examples of non-salutogenically focused categories of outcomes include a composite of infant morbidity outcomes (reported 141 times), maternal infection (fever, temperature, sepsis, etc) (reported 74 times), fetal death, neonatal loss or stillbirth (reported 65 times), neonatal admission to NICU/SCBU (reported 49 times), labour and/or birth trauma (reported 32 times) and induction and/or labour augmentation (artificial rupture of membranes/oxytocin) (reported 29 times). These findings, without suggesting that adversity is not an important measure of maternal health, demonstrate a lack of support for a salutogenic approach to measuring health and wellbeing in maternity care research. Rather, the findings of the review reinforce the dominant focus on risk reduction that abounds in clinical maternity practice and policy (Royal College of Midwives, 2005) with significantly less consideration given to outcome measures that are reflective of maternal and neonatal health and wellbeing. Our systematic review of reviews concludes by suggesting that this

> *... paucity of salutogenically-focused outcomes has implications for maternity care research in that the avoidance of ill-health or adversity remains the key driver for measuring the effectiveness of interventions. Adopting a more salutogenically-focused approach to maternity care research by incorporating salutogenically-focused outcome measures... has the potential to provide evidence on women's... well-being and on their sense of coherence... It will allow for positive measures of maternal health to be identified and perhaps clarify more easily, in the context of the comparative effects of maternity care interventions, which interventions are promotional of positive health and well-being.* (Smith *et al*, 2014: 155)

The review presents a first step in developing a COS of salutogenically focused outcome measures for use in studies in intrapartum maternity care intervention research. We believe that developing a minimum COS of these outcomes will provide outcome measures that are reflective of positive maternal health and will thus support a move away from the dominant focus on adversity in research. Using the 16 categories of identified outcomes, with an option for providing two further outcomes not contained in the list, an electronic Delphi survey is planned to achieve international key stakeholder consensus on a minimum final set of salutogenic intrapartum core outcomes (SIPCO). When finalised, we would encourage researchers in maternity care to consider use of SIPCO, in trials, systematic reviews, and other studies, on intrapartum maternity care.

Core outcome sets in maternity care: where are we?

The absence of COS for use in maternity care research is problematic for evidence determination and synthesis. Developing COS for specific conditions in maternity care would help overcome variation in outcomes measured across studies, reduce over-selection of outcomes in studies and non-reporting of outcomes, and reduce potential outcome reporting bias. Work in developing COS in maternity care has begun (Table 2) and is gaining momentum (Table 3); however, as seen in the limited number of complete and planned projects, we have some way yet to go.

Table 2:

Examples of published reports on COS-specific or COS-related projects in maternity care

STUDY	TITLE	AIM	METHODS	RESULTS
Devane *et al* (2007)	Evaluating maternity care: a core set of outcome measures	To identify a minimum set of outcome measures to evaluate models of maternity care	International eDelphi survey	A final minimum set of 48 outcomes for use in research on models of maternity care identified (see Box 1)
Begley *et al* (2014)	Outcome measures in studies on the use of oxytocin for the treatment of delay in labour: a systematic review	To identify primary and secondary outcome measures in randomised trials, and systematic reviews of randomised trials, measuring the effectiveness of oxytocin for treatment of delay in the first and second stages of labour	Systematic review	28 studies and 5 systematic reviews; a total of 23 outcomes were used in two or more studies or reviews; caesarean section was the most frequently measured primary outcome; other commonly reported outcomes in descending order included length of labour, measurements of uterine activity and mode of vaginal birth
Smith *et al* (2014)	Salutogenically focused outcomes in systematic reviews of intrapartum interventions: a systematic review of systematic reviews	To identify salutogenically focused outcomes reported in systematic reviews of intrapartum interventions	Systematic review of systematic reviews	102 reviews; 16 categories of salutogenically focused outcomes identified compared to 49 categories of non-salutogenically focused outcomes
Meher & Alfirevic (2014)	Choice of primary outcomes in randomised trials and systematic reviews evaluating interventions for preterm birth prevention: a systematic review	To systematically review the choice and consistency of primary outcomes in trials and systematic reviews of interventions for preventing preterm birth	Systematic review	103 trials and 33 systematic reviews; 72 different primary outcomes were reported in 103 trials; 29 different primary outcomes were reported in 33 systematic reviews; there is a considerable lack of consistency in the choice of outcomes in research on preterm birth

Examples of conditions in maternity care targeted for future COS development

TITLE	DESCRIPTION	STATUS
A core outcome set for very preterm birth*	A preliminary meeting of clinicians, service users and researchers was held at the 2nd COMET meeting in July 2011; a James Lind Alliance partnership for setting research priorities and to discuss the opportunities to initiate discussions about core outcome sets for very preterm birth	Ongoing
Core outcomes for studies on prevention of preterm birth in high-risk women: COPOP project*	The objective of this project is to develop a COS for studies focusing on prevention of preterm birth in high-risk population. The target population is pregnant woman with a high risk for preterm birth (defined as having a history of preterm birth and/or short cervix) and their offspring (neonatal and childhood period)	
A core outcome set for hypertensive disorders in pregnancy*	The aim is to produce, disseminate, and implement a core outcome set for hypertensive disorders in pregnancy.	Ongoing
Core outcomes for clinical trials in pregnant women with epilepsy*	To develop a COS for clinical trials on the management of epilepsy in pregnant women. Objectives: 1. To perform a systematic literature review to produce a comprehensive list of all maternal and neonatal outcomes reported in recent studies of pregnant women with epilepsy 2. To use the Delphi technique to refine the outcome list into a COS agreed by key stakeholders	Commenced (under peer review)
Core outcomes for clinical trials in gestational diabetes**	To develop a COS for use in clinical trials, and other studies, for the screening, prevention and treatment of gestational diabetes, and, where relevant, to define methods for measuring the outcomes included in this set	Planned for 2017
Core outcomes for clinical trials in pre-eclampsia**	To develop a COS for use in clinical trials in the prevention and treatment of pre-eclampsia	Commenced

*Identified from the COMET database (www.comet-initiative.org)

**Identified through personal communication

Three systematic reviews listed in Table 2 (Meher & Alfirevic, 2014; Begley *et al*, 2014; Smith *et al*, 2014) do not actually provide final COS, rather, they support the need for the development of COS. The study by Devane *et al* (2007) is the only study we could identify that provides a final COS for use on a maternity care topic. In this study, a three-round electronic Delphi was used to achieve international consensus on a minimum final set of outcomes for use in evaluating models of maternity care. The Delphi method is well suited to consensus building as it involves the distribution of a series of questionnaires to a panel of experts, such as service users and appropriate others, on the topic under investigation. Following each round, the results are analysed and items receiving ratings of importance (based on various rating scales as selected for the study) are forwarded to the next round for further rating. Items judged to be important (or rated highly) on the final round are deemed those on which consensus has been achieved. Participants in the Devane *et al* (2007) consensus exercise (n=152 completing all three rounds) were from key stakeholder groups and included women as maternity service users, midwives, obstetricians, paediatricians / neonatologists, policy-makers, and service providers and researchers with expertise in maternity care. The final minimum outcome set consists of 48 outcomes (Box 1).

Box 1:

COS for evaluating models of maternity care (Devane *et al*, 2007)

- Maternal death (the death of a woman while pregnant or within 42 days of termination of pregnancy)
- Mode of birth (e.g., spontaneous vaginal, forceps, vaginal breech, caesarean section, vacuum extraction)
- Neonatal death (death before the age of 28 completed days after live birth)
- Stillbirth (a fetal death in late pregnancy)
- Type of labour onset (manner in which labour started, i.e., induced, spontaneous, planned caesarean section)
- Neonatal admission to special care and/or intensive care unit
- Birth injury to infant
- Ruptured uterus
- Postpartum haemorrhage (excess blood loss from the birth canal after childbirth)

- Mother requires admission to intensive care
- Maternal postnatal readmission to hospital
- Method of infant feeding
- Vaginal birth after previous caesarean section (VBAC)
- Gestational age at birth
- Postnatal depression
- Place of birth
- Neonatal resuscitation required
- Normal (i.e., physiological) birth without intervention (vaginal birth without induction, episiotomy, or epidural)
- Oxytocin augmentation of labour (drug used to assist progress of labour)
- Anal sphincter damage
- Hypoxic ischemic encephalopathy (a condition of injury to the brain)
- Intrapartum hypertensive disorders of pregnancy (a group of diseases characterised by high blood pressure with or without proteinuria; this group includes pre-eclampsia, eclampsia, and the syndrome of HELLP)
- Hypertensive disorders of pregnancy (a group of diseases characterised by high blood pressure with or without proteinuria; this group includes pre-eclampsia, eclampsia, and the syndrome of HELLP)
- Puerperal psychosis (a mood disorder often accompanied by features such as loss of contact with reality, hallucinations, severe thought disturbance, and abnormal behaviour)
- Maternal faecal incontinence
- Birth asphyxia (occurs when a baby does not receive enough oxygen before, during, or just after birth)
- Breastfeeding at discharge
- Neonatal readmission to hospital
- Apgar score at 5 minutes
- Trial of labour after previous caesarean delivery
- Breastfeeding at 3 months
- Maternal satisfaction (postnatal)
- Infant birth weight
- Neonatal fitting/seizures
- Infant requiring intubation
- Congenital anomaly (chromosomal, genetic, and/or structural)
- Use of pharmacological analgesia/anaesthesia (e.g., Entonox, epidural, pethidine)
- Maternal satisfaction (antenatal)
- Postnatal hypertensive disorders of pregnancy (a group of diseases characterised by high blood pressure with or without proteinuria; this

group includes pre-eclampsia, eclampsia, and the syndrome of HELLP)
- Maternal satisfaction (intrapartum)
- Caesarean section wound infection
- Pulmonary embolism (a condition in which a blood clot that has formed elsewhere in the body travels to the lungs)
- Intrauterine growth restriction (commonly used when the birthweight is at or below the 10th percentile for gestational age and sex)
- Preterm labor (onset of labor before 37 completed weeks of pregnancy)
- Meconium aspiration (means the newborn inhales a mixture of meconium and amniotic fluid, either in the uterus or just after delivery)
- Intrapartum haemorrhage (excessive blood loss from the birth canal during labour)
- Neonatal infection
- Shoulder dystocia

It is important to note that some of these outcomes may only occur after 28 or even 42 days after birth. This demonstrates that, in developing a COS for use in maternity care, there is some dependency on the timing of the assessment of an outcome. Focusing on outcomes at or directly after birth limits the view of what matters in the postpartum period or even later in life. A discussion on the timing of assessing COS in maternity care is therefore warranted.

Core outcome set development: the COMET Initiative and others

COS for research in health conditions are needed and will be beneficial, and it does appear that this need is increasingly being recognised and attended to as reflected in the considerable growth of COS-related publications year on year (Gargon *et al,* 2014). With this comes the need for accurate and robust methods for COS development. The COMET (Core Outcomes Measures in Effectiveness Trials) Initiative was established in 2010. This initiative is focusing on methods for developing and implementing COS. A recent systematic review, however, on choosing important outcomes for comparative effectiveness research, performed by members of the COMET team (Gargon *et al,* 2014), demonstrated variation in methods that are currently being used to develop COS (Table 4). Variation in methods for development presents its own problems in that researchers who wish to use COS need to be reassured that these COS have been developed using methodologically sound and robust methods and that the COS are valid and reliable. Work to standardise and develop robust methods for developing COS is currently ongoing within the COMET Initiative.

Table 4:
Main methods used to develop COS (Gargon *et al*, 2014)

METHOD	NO. OF STUDIES USING METHOD (N=198)
Mixed methods	74
Semi-structured group discussion only	57
Unstructured group discussion only	18
No methods described	16
Consensus development conference only	12
Literature/systematic review only	11
Delphi only	6
Survey only	3
Nominal Group Technique only	1

Other groups as well as COMET are also interested and involved in COS activity. A detailed discussion on these is outside the scope of this chapter; rather, Box 2 lists some of these groups and provides the links to their websites. One initiative listed in Box 2 that does warrant further mention, as it is connected strongly to maternity care, is the CoRe Outcomes in WomeN's health (CROWN) Initiative (www.crown-initiative.org). This initiative involves the coming together of the editors of over 70 women's health journals to support and encourage the development of COS in women's health. The strategic aims of CROWN are:

> *1) Form a consortium among all gynaecology-obstetrics and related journals to promote core outcome sets in all areas of our specialty; 2) Encourage researchers to develop core outcome sets using robust consensus methodology involving multiple stakeholders, including patients; 3) Strongly encourage the reporting of results for core outcome sets; 4) Organise robust peer-review and effective dissemination of manuscripts describing core outcome sets; 5) Facilitate embedding of core outcome sets in research practice, working closely with researchers, reviewers, funders and guideline makers*
> (Khan, 2014: 1181).

CROWN, while recently established and likely to expand and develop further, does currently provide an important impetus for developing COS specifically in women's health, including COS for maternity care conditions. CROWN presents a women's health-specific resource and, complemented by COMET, may provide valuable informative and advisory support for those interested in developing COS for use in maternity care research.

Box 2:

Additional groups involved in COS development

- Outcome Measures in Rheumatology (OMERACT) (www.omeract.org)
- Harmonising Outcome Measures for Eczema (HOME) (www.homeforeczema.org)
- CoRe Outcomes in WomeN's health (CROWN) (www.crown-initiative.org)
- WOMen and Babies health and wellbeing: Action through Trials (WOMBAT) (www.wombatcollaboration.net)

Initiatives such as COMET and CROWN predominantly or exclusively focus on 'what' to measure. There are simultaneously and collaboratively other groups who are focusing on methods of 'how' to measure outcomes, and it is important that future COS developers are aware of these. Standardising how an outcome should be measured is an essential second step in successful implementation of a COS. One such initiative is the COnsensus-based Standards for the selection of health Measurement Instruments (COSMIN) (www.cosmin.nl/cosmin). The strategic aim of COSMIN is to improve the selection of health measurement instruments for use in studies on a specific condition, so that standardised, valid and reliable instruments might be used. In achieving their aim, COSMIN have developed a critical appraisal checklist that provides researchers with standards for evaluating the methodological quality of studies on the measurement properties of health measurement instruments; for example, performance-based instruments or clinical rating scales. The checklist was developed using robust methods involving international collaboration with experts and an international Delphi study. In addition to its use in primary studies, the COSMIN checklist can also be used in evaluating the methodological quality of studies on measurement properties in systematic reviews of measurement properties and as a guide when designing or reporting on a study of measurement properties. Furthermore, reviewers or editors of healthcare journals can use the checklist to appraise the methodological quality of submitted studies on measurement properties and to check whether all important design aspects and statistical methods have been clearly reported. The COSMIN checklist can be accessed and downloaded using the following link: www.cosmin.nl/cosmin-checklist_8_0.html.

Conclusion

The focus of this chapter was on core outcomes in maternity care research. Through discussion and evidence from surveys, and other reports, the extent of outcome variation and outcome reporting bias in research in maternity care was highlighted. A lack of current COS for use in maternity care was also noted. While some work has been completed, and other work is ongoing, only one final minimum COS for use in maternity care was identified (Devane *et al*, 2007) and this COS was developed for evaluating models of maternity care. This demonstrates a clear and urgent need for the development of COS for use across a multitude of conditions that form the basis for research in maternity care. The COMET and CROWN Initiatives are some such groups that have been purposively established to explore COS and assist by providing support and advice to those who are interested in COS development and implementation. We encourage anyone interested in developing a COS for any condition in maternity care to consider contacting and engaging with these groups. To quote from the CROWN home page (www.crown-initiative.org):

> *We are coming together to address the widespread, unwarranted variation in reporting of outcomes. This problem makes comparison between and combination of results across studies difficult, if not impossible. As a result there can be difficulties in synthesising evidence to generate recommendations for clinical practice which is detrimental to the health of women and their babies.*

COS have the potential to optimise the health and wellbeing of women and babies. With maternity care research prolific on a global scale, the development of COS for use in research is timely and necessary.

References

Begley CM, Gross MM, Dencker A, Benstoem C, Berg M & Devane D (2014). Outcome measures in studies on the use of oxytocin for the treatment of delay in labour: A systematic review. *Midwifery* 30: 975-982.

Clarke M (2007). Standardising outcomes for clinical trials and systematic reviews. *Trials* 8: 39.

Devane D, Begley CM, Clarke M, Horey D & OBoyle C (2007). Evaluating maternity care: a core set of outcome measures. *Birth* 34(2): 164-172.

Dickersin K, Chan S & Chalmers TC (1987). Publication bias and clinical trials. *Control Clin Trials* 8(4): 343-353.

Dwan K, Altman DG, Arnaiz JA, Bloom J, Chan A, Cronin E, Decullier E, Easterbrook PJ, Von Elm E, Gamble C, Ghersi D, Ioannidid JPA, Simes J & Williamson PR (2008). Systematic review of empirical evidence of study publication bias and outcome reporting bias. *PLoS ONE* 3(8): e3081.

Dworkin RH, Turk DC & Wyrwich KW (2008). Interpreting the clinical importance of treatment outcomes in chronic pain clinical trials: IMMPACT recommendations. *J Pain* 9(2): 105-121.

Gargon E, Gurung B, Medley N, Altman DG, Blazeby JM, Clarke M & Williamson PR (2014). Choosing important health outcomes for comparative effectiveness research: a systematic review. *PLOS ONE* 9(6):1-12.

Hutton JL & Williamson PR (2000). Bias in meta-analysis due to outcome variable selection within studies. *Applied Statistics* 49: 359-370.

Khan K on behalf of Chief Editors of Journals participating in The CROWN Initiative (2014). The CROWN Initiative: journal editors invite researchers to develop core outcomes in women's health. *BJOG* 121: 1181-1182.

Kirkham JJ, Dwan KM, Altman DG, Gamble C, Dodd S, Smyth R & Williamson PR (2010). The impact of outcome reporting bias in randomized controlled trials on a cohort of systematic reviews. *BMJ* 340: C365.

Meher S & Alfirevic Z (2014). Choice of primary outcomes in randomized trials and systematic reviews evaluating interventions for preterm birth prevention: a systematic review. *BJOG* 121: 1188-1196.

Miyar J & Adams CE (2012). Content and quality of 10000 controlled trials in schizophrenia over 60 years. *Schizophr Bull* 39(1): 226-9.

Royal College of Midwives (2005). Rebirthing midwifery. *RCM Midwives* 8(8): 346-349. Available from: www.rcm.org.uk/midwives/features/rebirthing-midwifery

Smith V, Daly D, Lundgren I, Eri T, Benstom C & Devane D (2014). Salutogenically focused outcomes in systematic reviews of intrapartum interventions: A systematic review of systematic reviews. *Midwifery* 30: e151-e156.

Smith V, Clarke M, Williamson PR & Gargon E (2015). Survey of new 2007 and 2011 Cochrane reviews found 37% of pre-specified outcomes not reported. *J Clin Epidemiol* 68(3): 237-245.

Smith V & Clarke M (2014). *Survey of outcomes in Cochrane Reviews: Pregnancy and Childbirth Group.* Paper presented at the Optimising Childbirth in Europe conference, April 9-10, 2014, Brussels, Belgium.

Smyth RMD, Kirkham JJ, Jacoby A, Altman DG, Gamble C & Williamson PR (2010). Frequency and reasons for outcome reporting bias in clinical trials: interviews with trialists. *BMJ* 341: C7153.

The COMET Initiative (2014). Available from: www.comet-initiative.org

Thornley B & Adams C (1998). Content and quality of 2000 controlled trials in schizophrenia over

50 years. *BMJ* 317: 1181-1184.

Turk DC, Dworkin RH & Allen RR (2003). Core outcome domains for chronic pain clinical trials: IMMPACT recommendations. *Pain* 106: 337-345.

Williamson PR, Altman DG, Blazeby JM, Clarke M, Devane D, Gargon E & Tugwell P (2012). Developing core outcome sets for clinical trials: issues to consider. *Trials* 13: 132.

Williamson PR & Clarke M (2012). The COMET (Core Outcome Measures in Effectiveness Trials) Initiative: its role in improving Cochrane Reviews [editorial]. *Cochrane Database of Systematic Reviews* 5: ED000041.

Wuytack F, Smith V, Clarke M, Williamson P & Gargon E (2015). Towards core outcome set (COS) development: a follow-up descriptive survey of outcomes in Cochrane reviews. *Systematic Reviews* 4(73): 1-9.

CHAPTER 4

Capturing the complexity of practice as an insider: in-labour ethnography

Jette Aaroe Clausen and Mário JDS Santos

> *Methods are not a way of opening a window on the world, but a way to interfere with it.*
>
> (Mol, 2002: 155)

Introduction

The vast majority of maternity care research is undertaken within the positivist paradigm, using quantitative methods to gather evidence. Current normal science thinking (Kuhn, 1962) constructs an evidence hierarchy in which systematic reviews of randomised controlled trials are at the top (Clausen, 2011; Downe, 2010). Much of this research has generated beneficial changes in maternity services, and improved wellbeing for women, babies, and families. However, it is unable to answer many of the complex (so called 'wicked') problems of practice that remain:

> *On the high ground, manageable problems lend themselves to solution through the application of research method and theory... In the swampy lowland, messy confusing problems defy technical solution... [these are]... the problems of greatest human concern* (Schön, 1983: 14).

The underlying logic that defines the current evidence hierarchy norm is based on the assumption that there is one single truth to be found for any question that might be asked and that, to find it, bias can and should be controlled using experimental methods. In contrast, social scientists and others working in the interactionist and constructivist paradigm maintain that human notions and experiences of reality are socially constructed (Berger & Luckman, 1966). Some highlight the contributions that non-human actors (i.e., laboratory instruments, concepts and organisations, to name a few) play in the research process (Latour, 1987). Once an experiment is set up, some potential outcomes come into focus, and others are rendered impossible (Berg & Timmermans, 2000). Framing a research question is not, therefore, an innocent act. Even as we state our research question, we frame the solutions we are allowed to imagine (Clausen, 2010).

Ethnography is a complex method of *reflexively* studying what people do and say, and the context in which this happens, usually over a long period of time (Hammersley & Atkinson, 1995). Since the early periods of the discipline, anthropologists travelled to faraway and exotic places in an attempt to describe the *unfamiliar* in *familiar* terms. Branislow Malinowski presented *Argonauts of the Western Pacific* in 1922, based on his fieldwork with the traditional societies of Papua New Guinea and the Trobiant Islands, and it was a landmark publication in both anthropology and ethnography. Since then, the advantages and disadvantages of studying familiar settings have been extensively discussed across disciplinary fields. In 1943, the urban sociologist William Foote Whyte published *Street Corner Society – The Social Structure of an Italian Slum*. Beyond its direct results, the work of William Foote White gave relevant insights into the shifting roles of the participant observer, who is neither completely an insider nor an outsider. Although not completely consensual (Becker, 1996), different modalities of ethnography, including multi-sited ethnography, on-line ethnography, auto-ethnography, and even multispecies ethnography, both in familiar or unfamiliar settings, are now used with a wide degree of academic and scientific acceptance. Nevertheless, up until recently, only a few social scientists have chosen the hospital as their field of research, despite its potential for the analysis of its organisation, its structure, its 'internal' culture and the particular features of the interactions between an array of social actors (Carapinheiro, 1993; Long, Hunter & van der Geest, 2008).

In terms of maternity care, the ethnographic method offers the possibility of exploring everyday birthing practices as they are performed. In healthcare settings, 'complexity, uncertainty and mess' enclose the potential to establish the connection between different theoretical and disciplinary backgrounds (Heat, 2013). This allows for an examination that goes beyond taken-for-granted understandings of everyday practices.

The aim of this chapter is to explore the under-researched area of health professionals doing *in-labour ethnography*. The analysis is based on two different experiences from the authors as they undertook their research on the labour ward, while also being a qualified midwife or undertaking clinical practice as a nurse. *In-labour ethnography* is thus invested with a double sense in this chapter. It includes the broad sense of in-labour as in the researcher's real work settings as participant observers, and the specific sense of in-labour as in intrapartum research. A health professional that elects ethnography as the methodology for researching a clinical setting is confronted with a complex context framed by professional responsibilities, unclear definitions of private and public spaces, shifting relations mediated by technology, and patient and professional plural expectations towards the ethnographer. As such, this chapter proposes a reflection on both the productive and on the problematic features of in-labour ethnography, although highlighting the value of this strategy.

In the first part of the chapter, we discuss the implications of being an insider doing ethnography in our own backyard, and the 'labour' of constructing a field site. In the second part of the chapter, we use a specific fieldwork example to frame a reflection on the productive features of in-labour ethnography as well as the challenges. Finally we strive to draw some conclusions from a debate that is far from consensual and concluded.

Complexity and the value of in-labour ethnography

Childbirth is a complex event and can be a life-changing experience for parents. It can be understood as a physiological phenomenon, but also in multiple other ways. These include the personal, biological (and microbiological), familiar, professional, organisational, political, spiritual, health, cultural and social. The recognition of this complexity implies the need to explore birth with different scientific methods, and to consider the added value of transdisciplinary approaches (Byrne & Callaghan, 2013).

Scholars from several disciplines have made highly relevant contributions to the understanding of the complexity within contemporary childbirth. However, the specific study of childbirth practices is a latecomer to the social studies of health and medicine, compared to other research topics (Clausen, 2014; Santos, 2014). It can be said that, until the mid 1970s, maternity care and childbirth were scarcely studied critically and as a phenomenon in its own right, remaining as a mere variable or operational concept (Macintyre, 1980). It seems that the social complexity of childbirth only started to be addressed following the theoretical positioning that emerged with second-wave feminism (Cova, 2005). There are many examples and we can only mention a few, which stand out for their pioneering efforts and the use of an ethnographic approach: Brigitte Jordan, who has been called the mother to the anthropology of childbirth for her seminal fieldwork around childbirth practices in Mexico, the USA, Sweden and the Netherlands in the late 20th century (see, among others, Jordan, 1997); and the sociologist Ann Oakley, who has worked on the transition to motherhood and on medicine as an institution of social control (see, for example, Oakley, 1980). These and other following scholars, crossing disciplinary borders, have promoted the integration of multiple views and transdisciplinary approaches which have helped to unveil the complex systems around childbirth.

Being an insider

Yet, medical science and evidence-based medicine are disciplines striving to belong to what Sharon Traweek (1988) has called *the culture of no culture*, i.e., a community sharing the conviction that science is *not* cultural. Evidence-based medicine subscribes to the ideal of a distant and detached researcher who explores a pre-existing world and a pre-defined practice. These research methods can be productive when asking about the *effect* of an intervention, but they allow us to explore only a very limited fragment of what is relevant to knowing about health and healthcare.

Scholars from the social sciences have helped to develop a strong argument around the productive and valid knowledge emerging from research projects that use ethnographic methods (Long, Hunter & van der Geest, 2008). However, Vered Amit (2000) stresses that a field site is not lying out there. To Amit, a field site comes into being as a consequence of the research process; it is constructed as a consequence of both hard work and circumstances:

> *...in a world of infinite interconnections and overlapping contexts, the ethnographic field cannot simply exist, awaiting discovery. It has to be laboriously constructed, prised apart from all other possibilities for contextualisation to which the constituent relationship and construction is inescapably shaped by the conceptual, professional, financial and relational*

opportunities and resources available to the ethnographer (Amit, 2000: 6).

However, the specificity of ethnography in hospital settings as a methodology is, as yet, understudied (Wind, 2008). Doing research in a hospital without being a health professional can be a difficult task to perform, implying a considerable amount of time, especially at the beginning of the research, before the presence of the researcher can be acceptable for patients and professionals. The argument of patient privacy has been frequently raised as a barrier to the presence of the observer and the publication of results (Oosterhoff, 2009). The mere existence of an outsider in the hospital's hierarchy, structure, and culture can be disquieting and uncomfortable, both for observers and observed, being in itself revelatory of particular dynamics of power and knowledge that circulate through different social actors (Carapinheiro, 1993), expressing in a particular way the notion of authoritative knowledge developed by Jordan (1997). As Wind (2008: 82) states, 'this lack of the possibility to participate more fully in an immersive capacity is intrinsic to most if not all hospital ethnography'. She proposes the concept of 'negotiated interactive observation' as a new definition of the participant observation at the hospital, encompassing the diversity of roles and the complexity of the setting, where *reflexivity* and *inter-subjectivity* seem to have offered only partial insight, so far (Wind, 2008: 84-7). In fact, it seems that, in-hospital ethnography, insider and outsider perspectives are entangled in order to achieve the development of new knowledge over a rather familiar context (Long, Hunter & van der Geest, 2008; Oosterhoff, 2009). Moreover, we argue that a professional background may, under the right circumstances, provide us with productive opportunities to know the field site that gives voice to valuable knowledge and practices that would otherwise be silenced:

> *[A] researcher must love their material to produce good research. Science studies researchers must get inside the science, learning to appreciate it with a passion of an insider. This is the mainly unrealised gift from anthropology to science studies. Immersion produces insight. Reifying theory as a higher life form gets in the way of love. Theory is a tool kit. We need to love our tools, as they help us do things not for themselves.* (Tsing, 2008: 1).

Tsing's view on the relationship between the researcher and the object of study is comparable to ethnomethodology. It suggests that being an insider is not a *hindrance* to develop research-based knowledge: it is the *sine qua non* of knowledge production. This also implies dealing with the tensions emerging from the dual role of active professional and participant observer, such as the 'frictions between insider and outsider perspectives; maintaining distance as opposed to being involved; and non-intervention versus intervention' (Oosterhoff, 2009: 258). More than considering the complexity of health settings, the challenge is to consider and explicitly take into account the complexity of relations established between the engaged ethnographer and the field site under construction.

In-labour ethnography – there is no room for the unengaged observer

Donna Haraway, a prominent scholar in feminist and science and technology studies, suggests the concept of *situated knowledge* as a way to frame questions about objectivity. She stresses that all scientific descriptions are *partial descriptions*. All scientific texts are produced by a human, a professional with a face, a body, an identity and a social position within the research settings and the wider society (Haraway, 1991). Jeanne Favret-Saada acknowledged that the researcher has an important role to play in the production of knowledge. She describes the fieldworker as someone who is situated in the field while becoming engaged in it. The study of witchcraft in France brought her to the realisation that there was no room for an *unengaged observer* (Favret-Saada, 1980). As she first started to ask questions about witches, she got no answers from her informants. The lack of answers was not a consequence of the informants' lack of knowledge; quite the contrary. By asking questions about witchcraft her informants began to identify her as a witch. It was simply *not* possible for an outside ethnographer to talk about witchcraft in order *only* to inform herself or her future readers. Talking about witchcraft was an act that also positioned Favret-Saada in a particular social space.

The researcher as 'an instrument' is a much-used metaphor in qualitative methodology. Rossman and Rallis (1998: 26) observe that this metaphor 'evokes an image of an antiseptic enterprise – one in which the researcher is merely a tool'. They suggest using the metaphor of '*a learner*', which is useful because it illuminates the fact that fieldwork is carried out in order to develop texts that will allow the researcher to talk about practices in new ways, transforming the unique situations experienced into intelligible knowledge, for an audience placed within or outside the field site. The relationship between a fieldworker and the informant carries difficulties and opportunities. In our view, this places an obligation on the researcher to be a present learner.

Researcher as stranger or homecomer

The need to be a present learner, and the impossibility of being an objective *tabula rasa* chimes with our own experiences. Even though we tried to ask naive questions during our fieldwork, our informants would seldom provide answers that could be understood by naive questioners. Instead, they would refer back to discussions relevant to the professional field that we all (researcher and researched) were familiar with. For example, those who knew that we knew the practices we studied prior to our research tended to make comparisons between *current* practices and draw lines to practices that had occurred in the *past*. It seems of crucial importance to acknowledge that informants take into account the background of the ethnographer when interacting and answering, and that this shapes the research relationship as well as the research products. Alfred Schuetz distinguished between the *homecomer* and the *stranger*. The stranger expects to come to an environment unknown to him:

> *[The] homecomer's attitude differs from that of the stranger. The latter is about to join a group which is not and never has been his own. He knows that he will find himself in an unfamiliar world, differently organised than that from which he comes, full of pitfalls and hard to master. The homecomer, however, expects to return to an environment of which he always had and – so he thinks – still has intimate knowledge and which he has just to take for granted in order to find his bearings within it. The approaching stranger has to anticipate in a more or less empty way what he will find; the homecomer has just to recur to the memories of his past* (Schuetz, 1945: 369).

According to Schuetz, life at home follows an organised pattern of routine. It has its well-determined goals and well-proved means to bring them about, consisting of traditions, habits, institutions and timetables for activities of all kinds (Schuetz, 1945). We both entered the field being already there, as members of the setting we studied and, as a consequence, we spoke the language of obstetrics and midwifery, and we knew many of the routines and problems those who work on a labour ward face in their daily activities. We were by no means innocent or able to claim that we were not involved with the field. However, we were also strangers – we had different particular knowledges and experiences from those (doctors, midwives, nurses) who worked on the wards we were researching in. Our hybrid identities as either 'nurse or midwife fieldworker' or as 'social scientist fieldworker' acted as productive positions from which we could develop an analysis that would provide an opportunity to disseminate and share knowledge that might, in turn, provide a basis from where we could discuss and even improve maternity care practices.

Positioning ourselves

Jette Aaroe Clausen is a Danish midwife, and a midwifery lecturer, with a PhD in science and technology studies. For her doctoral studies, she did ethnography in a labour ward where she had previously worked, in Denmark. Mário Santos is a Portuguese nurse who has also worked in an obstetric ward since the beginning of his career, in a private hospital in Portugal. He has been involved in postgraduate training, where he did an ethnographic exercise in his own workplace. He is currently a PhD candidate in sociology, researching home birth networks through multi-sited ethnography. When entering the field site, both were recognised with multiple identities. Many people knew the researchers as colleagues, with different degrees of familiarity; while to other actors present in the field, the researchers were unknown.

In fact, acording to Hammersley and Atkinson (1995), fieldworkers can, to some extent, take on different roles in the field. Personal relations and personal experience are often understood as being outside science, but here they are obviously, intrinsically connected. In Rayna Rapp's (1999) interesting and inspiring study, she describes how her own personal experience of carrying a child with Down's syndrome was used in a productive way in her study into amniocentesis. Furthermore, Tereso (2005), a nurse-midwife, on her ethnography in a labour ward, mentions how being known by professionals as a colleague, and being recognised by users as a professional had mostly a positive impact, as there was little resistance to the researcher's presence and an easy expansion of the field of observation to other areas of the labour ward. Indeed, it is arguable if this is an exceptional feature of particular scientific researches using ethnography, or if it is an overlooked condition of all research, to some degree, shaded for the sake of *variable control* and *scientificity*.

Oosterhoff (2009) gives us some systematic understanding of these connections based on her action-research project in Vietnam, where she dealt with the double role of a public health worker and a medical anthropologist:

> *Such dual roles offer practical advantages, for example having a natural relationship with colleagues and patients with whom one can regularly discuss research directions and ideas. It also provides action-focused researchers with an existing organizational and institutional context that can provide immediate support in terms of human resources, methods and tools for data collection [...]. It might allow for greater empathy, both with medical professionals and patients because it enables the researcher to better understand the context in which decisions are made. A joint working experience could help to establish 'intersubjectivity,' a shared cognition and consensus about the situation we study. However, it might increase the empathy with medical professionals at the cost of empathy with patients* (Oosterhoff, 2009: 264-5).

Nevertheless, Oosterhoff presents a slightly different experience from what we are aiming to discuss; which is worth clarifying, as it can produce different processes and relationships. Being a Dutch woman in Vietnam, she frequently felt like an *outsider*, althought she was an *insider* to the profession and the process she was researching. This is quite distinct from the in-labour ethnographic approach we are presenting here, where the familiarity with the setting and its actors is more significant.

Mário's and Jette's experiences have much in common, but have some relevant differences too. Similarly to Tereso and Oosterhoof, Mário's ethnographic exercise in the labour ward allowed him to quickly gain the formal permission to access the field, and to easily conquer the indispensable integration in the field as a researcher. On the other hand, it required a high degree of reflexivity and critical analysis of the changing setting, combined with the ability to register field notes, while maintaining his professional role as a nurse. This was not always successfully accomplished – the role of the nurse occasionally overruled the role of the researcher. Despite this, recognising the extraordinary out of the familiar was overwhelming. The differences in the name and the spatial organisation of the nurses' rooms (the *work* room) and the doctors' room (the *meetings* room), which were always there, could then be interpreted as denouncing a socially constructed distinction of the manual *versus* intellectual work of these professional groups. The frontier between insider and outsider was, in fact, diluted.

Jette's experience also illustrates the difficulties of taking on different roles. Even though Jette had worked within midwifery for more than 20 years, there were many situations during her fieldwork that seemed simple, but turned out to be complicated. Such situations often involved different kinds of *technology*, such as telephones and drip machines. Increasing the oxytocin drip (which starts or accelerates labour via an intravenous line) is an easy task for a midwife. However, the first time she got this request in her fieldwork setting, Jette realised that the interface on the relevant machine had changed since she was actively practising. What was once an easy task to perform had become much more complicated. When Jette was practising as a midwife the delivery of oxytocin was calculated by *drips* per minute. In the fieldwork situation, it was done by *millilitres* per minute, so every time the midwife asked Jette to increase the drip, she had to do a mental calculation, turning millilitres into drips, since, without doing so, she did not know if the requested increase was likely to be safe and effective. As an insider researcher, Jette could not just do what was requested of her without taking into account what her informants might think of her as a midwife, and thus that she was responsible for her actions in a different way to an ethnographer who was not a midwife would be.

Balancing hybrid identities during in-labour ethnography can thus provide challenging situations. In another example, Jette was in the office when a midwife had just read a suspicious trace on the fetal monitor. The usual practice was to summon a senior midwife and an obstetrician to the office, to get an overview of the situation before they talked to the woman. In this kind of situation, the decision had to be made quickly on whether to intervene or not. These decisions were often highly *distributed*. The midwife assigned to take care of the woman, the senior midwife and an obstetrician might discuss the trace, with other attending midwives joining in occasionally. Jette generally kept silent, but she was also wearing the green uniform of labour ward staff. Her verbal silence, along with the uniform, created an invisible presence, as a fieldworker, making her prone to be translated into *a midwife who supported a specific interpretation of a fetal heart rate*. It was important for her to avoid such interpretations of her (non) actions. In situations like this she chose to make her position clear to everybody present. However, the situation did not usually leave her much time to select a specific role, as decisions had to be made quickly when there was a concern about the wellbeing of the fetus. Jette would sometimes use *irony* as a strategy in this situation (Haraway, 2004: 7), something along the lines of 'I am happy that I am only a fieldworker, who does not need to take a stand on this trace.' This strategy was used to make a short statement that recognised her contradictory position as a fieldworker, while being a midwife, but also renouncing her midwife identity in the moment. She was hoping to achieve the position of someone who *was there without being there*.

For Jette, making this position explicit was important on ethical grounds. She could not accept that her mere silent presence would tip the reading of a trace in one or the other direction (intervention/wait and see). When she stepped forward and recognised herself as a fieldworker who did not need to take responsibility and decide how to act on the trace in situations like these, she actually came to bear witness to the difficulty that the professionals involved experienced. Being positioned as a midwife or an obstetrician meant that they had to decide on what to do, and they had to do it on the basis of the information that they had available in this situation. They also knew that what is right, now, can later be proven wrong. This is an often-present dilemma in clinical work. Births progress forward all the time, but the trace will be interpreted backwards, which sometimes produces different readings. As Latour (1987) notes, text (like fetal heart traces) is always in the hands of later users. On more than one occasion when Jette made her role known, some of the involved staff would reply 'you lucky one' or 'I wish it was me'. The message was clear: clinical work is filled with uncertainty, and as such it is a difficult place to be.

In-labouring: learning from Annegrethe's story

In this following section we selected an example from Jette's field notes and further analysis (Clausen, 2010: 36-7) to highlight how our previous involvement with the field and the dynamic of playing a double role in the particular setting of an obstetric ward have a potential impact on the outcome of our studies.

> *Annegrethe, a first-time mother, telephoned the ward and talked to a midwife because she had not felt her baby all day. The midwife had asked her*

to come in to run a trace. Annegrethe is now lying in the admitting room across the hallway, and she has a fetal monitor attached to her stomach. The trace of the fetal heart can simultaneously be observed on a screen in the midwives' office, but this trace is particularly difficult to read. It's not pathological but it's not normal either; it lacks sufficient variation in its baseline. This can be a bad sign, but it can also be benign; it can be difficult to distinguish between a baby in distress and a sleeping baby. I feel a little stressed as I watched the trace. Does Eva, the midwife who I follow on this shift, see this? I can't see her anywhere, and I start to wonder why Eva isn't checking on this woman. She knows that she [Annegrethe] did not feel her baby moving. I start asking myself, 'am I responsible here?' Had I been on duty as a midwife, there would not have been doubt in my mind and I would have attended to this woman immediately. Now, as a fieldworker, I am in doubt. What's the right thing to do?

My identity as a fieldworker does not allow me to attend to the woman on my own, so I remain in the office and, while I wait, I keep an eye on the monitor. Another midwife, Anne turns up and she says: "What is this? Hasn't somebody called a doctor?" I feel trapped. The trace makes me feel slightly uneasy, on the other hand I think that calling for a doctor is an overreaction, and I don't want to be disloyal to Eva either. 'I don't think it can wait,' says Anna as she picks up the phone. At the same moment, Eva steps into the office and asks 'What is going on here?' I can see that she feels offended. 'It's a sleeping baby; our guidelines say that a trace like that is normal if it doesn't extend for half an hour. Give it some time.' The attention of a group of midwives who overhear this conversation is drawn to the trace. Their attention is brought about by the discussion of the trace rather than the pattern of the trace itself.

Before I know it, we are four people standing right next to Annegrethe, all watching the trace. The senior midwife starts to palpate her stomach. She wants to see if the baby reacts to stimulation. While she works she addresses the baby 'It's time to wake up, we want to see that you can kick.' It's an extremely busy shift, and a doctor arrives in the room, but she steps back as she watches the senior midwife at work. After a while the heart trace looks slightly different and the senior midwife turns to the doctor and says 'The caesarean is in ward two, we need to hurry now.' It's not Annegrethe that she refers to, but another woman who has been admitted because she is in preterm labour. Then she turns to me. 'Jette you have to work now.

I need Anne to go with me. You stay in here 'till that trace is normal.' I see hesitation in her face, and she stresses 'I want to see at least three accelerations before you take the belts off. Give me three accelerations.' As she speaks she underlines three, with her fingers. I stay and they all leave. I feel slightly uneasy towards the woman. How does she experience this situation? She knows that I am a fieldworker, and now she is left with me.

I felt obliged to offer some kind of explanation, so I say 'I know I introduced myself as someone who does research in this department, but you should know that I am also a midwife; that's why the senior midwife asked me to stay with you. It's extremely busy tonight, and we need all the hands we can get.' The woman laughs. 'It's all right. I am a nurse. I work in the intensive unit here in Skejby. I know all about busy shifts and machines creating false alarms. It is ok with me.'

It was not only Jette who had multiple identities; the labouring women had them too. This made it easy to become a midwife in this situation. The role of a homecomer was productive here; it produced an opportunity to learn how fetal monitoring is enacted. Star and Strauss (1999) use the concept of deleted work to describe work that is normally not recognised and described. This situation provided Jette with an opportunity to learn about work that is not often spoken of.

The fact that it is the senior midwife who delegates this work to Jette is helpful. As a homecomer who has been away for some time, fetal heart rates are not part of everyday life as they were when Jette was a colleague to the senior midwife a long time ago. The senior midwife was aware of this, so she underlined what she wants: 'Give me three accelerations.' Jette could not do this on her own; she had to involve the woman, the fetus and the fetal monitor. This opened up a space where the researcher could be allowed to touch the woman as a midwife. Due to her midwifery background, Jette knew what to do in a situation like this; the senior midwife did not expect her to sit around and wait for three accelerations. If the trace did not change within a reasonable time, she would expect the researcher to do something. Midwives have different ways to produce accelerations: they can, for example, palpate the woman's abdomen in order to stimulate the fetus to move, or offer some cold water for the woman to drink, in order to make the fetus wake up. This incident brought to light how much deleted work it takes to produce acceptable traces. A trace is not simply produced by a passive monitoring of the fetal heart:

the production of an acceptable trace involves both women, fetuses, and midwives. This was a process which was not necessarily circumscribed to the procedure itself.

Being a midwife doing fieldwork came with difficulties but also with possibilities, because Jette's midwifery experience helped to get around difficult situations. In the situation described above, and in others, one could question: what would have happened if this child had been unexpectedly compromised when it was born? Would the reseacher be asked about what was observed during labour? And would she be asked for a midwifery opinion? Texts are always in the hand of later users as noted above (Latour, 1987). Could Jette have been asked to hand over the field notes, and in this process, would they be translated into a supplement to the woman's medical notes? In relation to a different but related clinical situation, Jette realised the need to stabilise her position as a fieldworker and destabilise her position as a midwife. In a meeting with the head of midwifery, Jette explained, without referring to specifics, that she had realised, while taking notes, that she might be asked to hand them over in cases of difficulty. As a researcher, Jette stated she could not do that, because it would compromise the confidentiality agreed with the observed staff. She understood the situation, and immediately wrote a letter before Jette left her office, stating that the notes were personal research notes and the department could not, in any circumstances, get access to these.

In *Ethnography Through Thick and Thin*, George Marcus (1997) introduces the concept of *complicity* to wisely describe how a productive ethnographer-informant relationship often requires the recognition, rather than the omission, of the outsideness of the ethnographer. He argues that there is a need for a new framing of this relationship, to encompass the way fieldwork is carried out today. Complicity is accomplished in an ethnographic relationship within the wider set of relationships that connect the researcher and their informants to 'specific sites elsewhere that affect their interactions (in relation to the influence of that «third»)' (Marcus, 1997: 122). Indeed, one of the aspects we highlight from these examples is the relevance and the productive potential of observers and observed acknowledging the specific features of the ethnographers – their background and insideness, but also their research agenda and their connections to other contexts and institutions – which position them culturally and socially as belonging to the outside world and, at the same time, contribute to building an image or a role for the ethnographers as having a place inside the hospital setting, as neither an insider nor an outsider.

Conclusion

The study of the complexity of pregnancy, childbirth and motherhood across disciplinary fields, and the relevant contribution of the social sciences, have equipped health professionals with theoretical and methodological tools for the critical and reflexive analysis of the healthcare settings where they practise and that they observe. The value of in-labour ethnography, we argue, is the capacity to bring to light social phenomena that would otherwise be undercovered or inaccessible to the common researcher. Managing the insideness and outsideness of the ethnographer, and making the way to the sweet spot of complicity, can be a challenging task. Nevertheless, the particular position of health professionals has a peerless potential to defy the way healthcare, and maternity care in particular, are viewed from inside the healthcare system. There is a transforming potential on the use of in-labour ethnography that health professionals should no longer undervalue.

References

Amit V (2000). Introduction - constructing the field. In: Amit V (ed), *Constructing the Field. Etnographic Fieldwork in the Contemporary World*. London: Routledge.

Becker H (1996). The epistemology of qualitative research. In: Jessor R, Colby A & Shweder RA (eds). *Ethnography and Human Development: Context and Meaning in Social Inquiry*, Chicago: University of Chicago Press.

Berg M & Timmermans S (2000). Orders and their others: on the constitution of universalities in medical work. *Configurations* 8 (1): 31-61. Available from: https://muse.jhu.edu/journals/configurations/v008/8.1berg.html

Berger PL & Luckmann T (1966). *The Social Construction of Reality – a Treatise in the Sociology of Knowledge*. Penguin Group.

Blumer H. (1986). *Symbolic Interactionism: Perspective and Method*. University of California Press .

Byrne D & Callaghan G (2013). *Complexity Theory: the State of the Art*. Taylor & Francis.

Carapinheiro G (1993). *Saberes e Poderes no Hospital – uma Sociologia dos Serviços Hospitalares* [Knowlege and power in the hospital – A sociology of hospital services]. Porto: Edições Afrontamento.

Casper M (1998). *The Making of the Unborn Patient – a Social Anatomy of Fetal Surgery*. New Brunswick , New Jersey, and London: Rutgers University Press.

Clausen JA (2010). How does materialty shape childbirth? An explorative journey into evidence, childbirth practices and science and technology studies (doctoral thesis). Aarhus, University of Aarhus.

Clausen JA (2011). RCTs and everyday practices ... a troubled relationship. In: Donna S (ed). *Promoting Normal Birth: Research, Reflections & Guidelines*. UK: Fresh Hearth Publishing, pp.127-138.

Clausen JA (2014). Childbirth practices. In: Cockerham WC, Dingwall R & Quah SR (eds.) *The Wiley-Blackwell Encyclopedia of Health, Illness, Behavior and Society*. Oxford: Blackwell Publishing.

Cova A (2005). Où en est l'histoire de la maternité? [What is the history of motherhood?] *Clio. Femmes, Genre, Histoire* 21: 189-211.

Downe S (2010). Beyond evidence-based medicine: complexity and stories of maternity care. *J Eval Clin Pract* 16(1): 232-237.

Duden B (1991). *The Woman beneath the Skin: a Doctor's Patients in Eighteenth-Century Germany*. Cambridge, Mass, and London: Harvard University Press.

Favret-Saada J (1980). *Deadly Words – Witchcraft in the Bocage*. Cambridge: Cambridge University Press.

Hammersley M & Atkinson P (1995). *Ethnography: Principles in Practice*. London: Routledge.

Haraway D (1991). Situated knowledges: the science question in feminism and the privilege of partial perspective. In: *Simians, Cyborgs and Women: The Reinvention of Nature*. London: Free Association Books.

Haraway D (2004). *The Haraway Reader*. New York: Routledge.

Heat I (2013). Complexity, uncertainty and mess as the links between science and the humanities in health care. In: Sturmberg JP & Martin C (eds). *Handbook of Systems and Complexity in Health*. Springer.

Jensen UJ (2006). Evidence, effectiveness and ethics: Cochrane´s legacy. In: Kristiansen IS & Mooney G (eds). *Evidence-Based Medicine in its Place*. London and New York: Frank Cass Publishers, pp20-32.

Jordan B (1997). Authoritative knowledge and its construction. In: Davis-Floyd R & Sargent CF (eds). *Childbirth and Authoritative Knowledge: Cross-Cultural Perspectives*. Berkeley and Los Angeles: University of California Press.

Kuhn TS (1962). *The Structure of Scientific Revolutions*. Chicago: The University of Chicago Press.

Latour B (1987). *Science in Action: How to Follow Scientists and Engineers through Society*. Massachusetts and Cambridge: Harvard University Press.

Long D, Hunter C & Van der Geest S (2008). When the field is a ward or a clinic: hospital ethnography. *Anthropol Med* 15(2): 71-78.

Macintyre S (1980). The sociology of reproduction. *Sociol Health Illn 2*(2): 215-222.

Marcus GE (1997). The uses of complicity in the changing mise-en-scène of anthropological fieldwork. *Representations* 59 (Special Issue: The Fate of "Culture": Geertz and Beyond), pp. 85-108. Available from: www.jstor.org/stable/2928816

Mol A (2002). *The Body Multiple: Ontology in Medical Practice*. Durham: Duke University Press.

Oakley A (1980) *Women Confined: Towards a Sociology of Childbirth*. Oxford: Martin Robertson.

Oakley A (2000). *Experiments in Knowing: Gender and Method in the Social Sciences*. Cambridge: Polity Press.

Oosterhoff P (2009). Observations on action research with HIV-positive women and state service providers in northern Vietnam. *Medische Antropologie* 21(2): 257-276. Available from: tma.socsci.uva.nl/21_2/oosterhoff.pdf

Rapp R (1999). *Testing Women, Testing the Fetus. The Social Impact of Amniocentesis in America*. New York: Routledge.

Rossman GB & Rallis SF (1998). *Learning in the Field. An Introduction to Qualitative Research*. London and New Delhi: SAGE Publications, Thousand Oaks

Santos M (2014). *Para uma sociologia da maternidade – um retrato temático da investigação sociológica portuguesa* [Towards a sociology of motherhood and maternity care – A thematic portrait of the Portuguese sociological research]. *CIES E-Working Papers*, (194/2014). Available from: http://cies.iscte.pt/np4/?newsId=453&fileName=CIES_WP194_Santos.pdf

Schön DA (1983). *The Reflective Practitioner: How Professionals Think in Action*. New York: Basic Books.

Schuetz A (1945). The homecomer. *Am J Sociol* 50(5): 369-376. Available from: www.jstor.org/stable/2771190

Star SL & Strauss A (1999). Layers of silence, arenas of voice: the ecology of visible and invisible work. *Computer Supported Cooperative Work (CSCW)* 8(1): 9-30.

Tereso A (2005). *Coagir ou Emancipar* [Coerce or emancipate]. Lisboa: Formasau.

Thomson C (2005). *Making Parents: The Ontological Choreography of Reproductive Technologies*. Cambridge: MIT Press.

Traweek S (1988). *Beamtimes and Lifetimes: The World of High Energy Physicists*. Cambridge, Massachusetts: Harvard University Press.

Tsing A (2008). Alien vs. predator. Presentation to the Danish Association for Science and Technology Studies' annual meeting June 6, 2008. *STS Encounters* 1(1). Available from: www.dasts.dk/wp-content/uploads/tsing-anna-2008-alien-vs-predator.pdf

Wind G (2008). Negotiated interactive observation: doing fieldwork in hospital settings. *Anthropol Med* 15(2): 79-89.

CHAPTER 5

Innovations in practice: challenges involved in knowledge transfer

Karin Minnie and Christa van der Walt

Introduction

All healthcare systems need an effective way to access the latest quality research as one mechanism to improve the quality of care across all levels of healthcare. Research spanning the past two decades indicates that individual health professionals find it challenging to keep abreast of the latest research findings. At the same time funders and researchers are under pressure to ensure that the findings of their research are shared with the relevant audiences as soon as possible. Findings of high-quality research cannot have an impact on the health of mothers and babies by the mere act of publication in research journals. There will be little or no impact if research findings are not translated into the 'language' of practitioners, managers and policy makers. In 1998 Schuster and colleagues reported that as many as 20-40% of patients do not receive care in accordance with principles based on the best scientific evidence and 20-25% of the care that they do receive is either not of any value or potentially harmful (Schuster *et al*, 1998). One can only speculate on the progress made since then.

The main purpose of this chapter is to discuss the challenges we, as a working group on knowledge transfer in a Cost Action study, faced in planning the knowledge transfer process for the multidisciplinary international research project.

Background

Within maternal-child health and the healthcare system in general, health professionals, scientists and policy makers are concerned about the increasing gap between the best available evidence and practice, and what actually transpires in practice and policy (World Health Organization, 2006; Cochrane *et al*, 2007; Lang *et al*, 2007). Recent figures indicate that the incubation period for original research to be incorporated into routine practice may be as long as two years. Unfortunately, this means that patients are not receiving the best possible care, and valuable resources might be wasted on inefficient, ineffective, and even harmful care (Alberta Health Services – Alberta Mental Health Board, 2009).

The concept of implementing research into practice is broad in scope, context dependent, complex, and encompasses all steps between the creation of knowledge and its application. It is in essence a two-way, interactive and iterative process.

What is knowledge transfer?

The first challenge encountered in planning for knowledge transfer was what Graham described as 'conceptual confusion' or 'terminology turmoil' (Graham, 2008).

This conceptual confusion was also evident in the working group's first discussion. Members from our working group on knowledge transfer have various scientific backgrounds, such as midwifery science, organisational and management sciences, economics and engineering. The team also had various degrees of experience and understanding of the concept of 'knowledge transfer'. The authors of this chapter, for example, follow the Canadian approach towards knowledge translation.

As the working group also planned to do a systematic review of knowledge transfer strategies, we first decided to do a rapid review to explore the various uses of the concept of knowledge transfer within the context of research. We started with a rapid evidence assessment and used a systematic search strategy using the following search terms: 'research' AND 'translation' OR 'transfer'.

As expected, we found an inconsistent use of terminology to refer to the transfer of research findings to practice such as knowledge transfer, sharing, translation, exchange, utilisation, implementation, diffusion, distribution and knowledge management. These terms are often used independently and interchangeably to refer to the transfer of research information between researchers and research users (health professionals, patients and policy makers). Many combinations such as 'research transfer', 'research utilisation', or 'knowledge utilisation' are found in publications. There is often a common overlap in the use of terms such as 'knowledge sharing', 'knowledge transfer', 'knowledge translation' and 'research' and 'knowledge dissemination' which complicates bibliographic searches.

The Canadian Institute of Health Research (2004) is of the opinion that knowledge translation includes knowledge dissemination, communication, technology transfer, ethical context, knowledge management, knowledge utilisation, a two-way exchange process between researchers and those who apply knowledge, implementation research, technology assessment, synthesis of results with the global context, and development of consensus guidelines.

Two major findings from the rapid review were that (1) knowledge transfer is embedded in knowledge management and used in managerial and organisational sciences, when referring to the transfer of best practices within organisations and between organisations; and (2) knowledge translation refers to the entire process as a collaborative effort between researchers and research users (practitioners and policy makers) and entails a two-way process. The task of our working team required strategies to transfer findings to various audiences. This process required a more linear approach.

It is therefore imperative that research teams ensure that they have a common understanding of the concept of 'knowledge transfer', taking into account the team members' subject field and frame of reference in terms of the terminology utilised by each member (Graham, 2008). Our team consisted primarily of researchers with a health background, who had some knowledge transfer experience. However, knowledge transfer was understood differently across the countries involved and also varied according to the level of experience of the team members. A better understanding of the meaning of knowledge transfer within the confusing landscape of semantics helped us to set the boundaries for our work.

The ultimate aim of knowledge transfer is uptake of knowledge with a clear impact on health professionals' behaviour, patient care outcomes, and cost-effectiveness. However, strategies to promote the implementation of knowledge were not included as we focused primarily on transferring the new knowledge to the relevant stakeholders and not on the implementation of it. We also excluded educational strategies aimed at undergraduate and postgraduate students to improve their knowledge of, for example, evidence-based practice. Finding a working definition of knowledge transfer resulted in a serious delay in the work of the knowledge transfer team.

After much debate during team meetings we reached a consensus to use the following working definition: knowledge transfer is the exchange, synthesis, and ethically-sound application of knowledge – with a complex system of interactions among researchers and users – to accelerate the capture of the benefits of research for the people we serve through improved health, more effective services and products, and a strengthened healthcare system.

Theoretical models of knowledge transfer

Eccles *et al* (2005: 107) suggest that researchers should position their knowledge translation/translation plans in a theory-based framework to guide the design, implementation and evaluation plans. Straus *et al* (2009) also speculate that theory-driven implementation will further the development of knowledge transfer by providing a framework which can facilitate an understanding of the change process and that can show which components were successful and which ones were not.

With the aforementioned lack of conceptual clarity of the concept of knowledge transfer, it is not a surprise that researchers found it challenging to develop a theory for knowledge transfer (Estabrooks, Thompson, Lovely & Hofmeyer, 2006). Lee and Garvin (2003), for example, critique the theoretical underpinning of knowledge transfer as mechanisms to disseminate knowledge as being embedded in a power relationship between decision makers, patients, health professionals and policy makers. This type of relationship often leads to resistance towards change. They suggest using a critical theoretical approach to focus on moving from information transfer to information exchange. This approach moves beyond a traditional one-directional flow of information to an exchange of information between researcher and research user.

Although there is no single model which is accepted as the norm by researchers worldwide, a range of theories, models and frameworks are available to guide researchers to plan for knowledge translation at individual, team, and organisational levels (Estabrooks *et al*, 2006; Eccles *et al*, 2005).

Different perspectives from the fields of organisational innovation, health, and social and behavioural sciences are helpful to understand the knowledge transfer process (Estabrooks *et al*, 2006; Straus *et al*, 2004). Social and behavioural theories can explain change and how it can be effected (Eccles *et al*, 2005), whereas social cognition theories suggest that audit and feedback is only an effective behavioural change intervention for motivated populations who agree that the change in behaviour is needed (Connor, 1998).

Einarson and Lockett (2006) emphasise the importance that information generated from research should reach the right people in the right format that works best for them. Traditional dissemination strategies primarily consist of the passive sharing of information knowledge and research findings. This is often done by means of in-service education, continuous professional education, conferences and publication in scientific journals. However, evidence to support the fact that these ways of sharing research findings actually have the required impact is lacking and the conclusion is that a different approach is required to bridge the gap between research findings and practice (Einarson & Lockett, 2006).

Understanding how knowledge is transformed into practice, or is adopted by research users, assisted knowledge transfer experts over the years to develop a number of knowledge transfer strategies and methods in order to effectively convey the core messages of research findings. Logan and Graham (1988) identified three basic knowledge transfer strategies, namely that of diffusion, dissemination and implementation. With reference to the practicalities of knowledge transfer, Goering (2005) identified four best practices for knowledge transfer, namely (1) research transfer and exchange planning; (2) excellent communication; (3) knowledge of the target audience; and (4) effective and strong linkage and exchange activities.

In the earlier work of Weiss (Weiss, 1979), five models of research utilisation from social science research were used to understand how knowledge is transferred into policy. This typology is still used by many researchers to guide their knowledge transfer plans. The Canadian Institute for Health Research is an example of an organisation which follows this model (Bennett & Jessani, 2011).

1. **Knowledge driven model/science push model/technical model**: This type of model is based on the assumption that if an idea / finding is good enough it will be used.
2. **Problem-solving model/demand-pull model/economic model**: The

direct application of the findings of research to solve a problem that was previously identified by the practitioner.

3. **Interactive model**: Policy makers seek information from a variety of sources, including social scientists, and the process of decision-making and research-to-policy dynamics involves interconnectedness and multiple-way exchanges.
4. **Political model**: The interests or opinions of policy makers predetermine the positions of policy makers and research is often used as 'ammunition' to support their position statements.
5. **Tactical model**: Research is not used for its content; rather the fact that it is being done is used by policy makers when pressed to take action on a particular issue.
6. **Enlightenment model**: Concepts and theoretical perspectives generated by social scientists permeate the policy-making process.

More recently the concept of knowledge translation (KT) became prominent, highlighting two concepts, namely that KT is part of the research process and requires a collaborative effort from researchers, research users (health professionals/practitioners/policy makers). An engaged relationship between researchers and practitioners, as users, is essential to communicate the meaning and potential use of research which in turn increases the impact of the findings of research on science and practice development (Duhamel, 2010). The value of the collaborative model for knowledge translation of Baumbusch *et al* (2008) is that it allows for research findings to be translated to align to the needs of the potential users and in such a way that it is meaningful to the users. This is the concept of 'knowledge exchange'. New knowledge should be packaged in such a way that the value of it is clear for knowledge users.

In improving the quality of healthcare, interventions need to function on four levels since different theories are needed to guide interventions at different levels of healthcare (Ferlie & Shortell, 2001). These levels are (1) the individual health professional, (2) healthcare groups or teams (communities of practice), (3) organisations providing healthcare, and (4) the larger healthcare system or environments where individual organisations are embedded. Theories of individual behaviour are more relevant to interventions targeting healthcare professionals as individuals, whereas organisational change theories are more relevant if interventions are directed at hospital or non-govermental organisation (NGO) levels (Eccles *et al*, 2005).

Eccles *et al* (2005) describe two ways to use theory to plan knowledge transfer. First, it is used to understand theory-based factors that underlie clinical practice in order to identify the processes or theoretical constructs that are important in current patterns of care and therefore should be the appropriate target of an implementation intervention. Secondly, theory can be used to develop and test interventions knowing which theoretical constructs are being targeted and design interventions to enhance the processes supporting change in such constructs.

In the COST project we aimed to transfer the findings of our research in such a manner that it would influence the behaviour of individual healthcare professionals, decision makers and policy makers. Packaging these messages is therefore important to address motivation, action and sustainability. For example, motivational theories explain how individuals reach the point where they decide to change or adapt their behaviour; action theories explain how individuals progress from intention to actual behavioural change; and stage theories propose an orderly progression through discrete stages toward behavioural change (Eccles *et al*, 2005). Finding suitable ways to 'package' these messages for different audiences is therefore important.

A framework for knowledge transfer

Lavis *et al* (2003) and Bennett and Jessani (2011) recommend an organising framework for a knowledge transfer strategy based on best available evidence. The five core questions within this framework are:

1. What should be transferred to decision makers? (the message)
2. To whom should research knowledge be transferred? (the target audience)
3. By whom should research knowledge be transferred? (the messenger)
4. How should research knowledge be transferred? (the knowledge transfer processes and supporting communication structure)
5. With what effect should research knowledge be transferred? (the evaluation)

Planning for knowledge transfer

Knowledge transfer strategies should be developed when a research project is conceptualised involving both researchers and research users, to collectively determine priorities, methods, interpretations of findings and dissemination strategies (Einarson & Lockett, 2006). Lavis *et al* (2003) warn researchers that not all research findings are transferrable and researchers should carefully consider 'take home messages'.

Developing a communication strategy

Communication is the cornerstone of effective knowledge transfer (Goering, 2005). The message(s) and knowledge transfer activities must be targeted to a specific audience. The organisations and individuals who deliver the message(s) must understand the audience and have a high level of credibility amongst members of a specific audience and of the knowledge transfer team. The message must also relate issues of concern within the target audience and must be based on rigorous research. Table 1 (on the next page) provides a valuable template to use for developing a communication strategy.

— To whom should the message be delivered?

When the researchers want to promote the latest findings to particular audiences according to the knowledge-driven model, it is essential that the message is formulated specifically for that audience. Again, an understanding of the audience is crucial (Jacobson *et al*, 2003), specifically as to their needs, preferences, current practices and readiness for change. At the same time researchers should know who are the opinion leaders, and champions for change, and also which audience should be targeted to successfully adopt the evidence. Researchers should also refrain from only targeting other researchers and include other audiences, such as practitioners, policy makers and managers of health institutions. Interaction with users, and understanding the context where research users come from and their needs related to new knowledge, are crucial requirements for effective knowledge transfer.

Table 1:

A communication strategy template (Bennett & Jessani, 2011)

Review	How have you been communicating in the past? What didn't work? What worked? How do you know?
Objectives	What do you want the communication to achieve? Are the objectives SMART? (Specific, measurable, achievable, realistic and timed)
Audience	Who is the audience? What information (and inspiration) do they need to act on your work? Who are opinion leaders in a given audience?
Message	What is the message? Do you have one message for multiple audiences or multiple messages for one or more audiences?
Basket	What kinds of communication 'products' (message packages) will best capture the messages? Why?
Channels	How will you promote and deliver the 'products'?
Resources	What is the available budget? Who may want to sponsor it? Will this change in the future? What communication hardware and skills do you have?
Timing	What is your timeline? Would a staged strategy, following stepwise interventions, be more appropriate? What special events or opportunities might arise? Does the work of like-minded organisations present ideas and opportunities?
Brand	Is all your communication "on brand?" How can you ensure that you are broadcasting the right message—consistently?
Feedback	Did your communication influence your audiences? How can you measure your performance and identify cause-effect clues between methods and results?

— By whom should the message be delivered?

This question will guide the researcher to identify the most credible 'messenger', both in the research group and the audience. Depending on the audience, academics and opinion leaders can be targeted to act as messengers. Bennett and Jessani (2011) recommend that the most credible person in the research team, usually the team leader, delivers the 'message' personally to the selected audiences.

— How should the message be delivered?

The question often asked is how the message should be 'packaged' to be effective. However, no single method has been demonstrated to be effective to transfer research findings into practice (Bennett & Jessani, 2011).

In the first place, the message should be relevant to the specific target group and should relate to a current concern. This principle highlights the importance of the relationship between researchers and the research users. Furthermore, the message should be clear, action-oriented and evidence-based. It must also be simple and specific for each target audience (Goering, 2005). A challenge for researchers is to move away from technical jargon, unnecessary words and acronyms towards using plain language that carries meaning to a specific target audience. Instead of presenting only the findings and conclusions, researchers should also transfer the bottom-line findings, and more specifically the recommendations of the findings, to practitioners, policy makers and managers. Lastly, researchers need to move beyond publication of their study in peer-reviewed journals as the main mechanism of dissemination, to an understanding that publication is only one way to transfer their findings.

Printed media is the medium most commonly used to transfer research findings to selected audiences. However, passive methods are less effective than interactive methods (Bennett & Jessani, 2011). Research publications and conference presentations only target a small audience and are seldom read by practitioners and policy makers. Face-to-face meetings with practitioners and one-pager briefs for policy makers have been shown to make a better impact on uptake of the research. However, researchers need to consider their budget when selecting the method of transfer.

The guiding principle is to know your audience and to know your message. The audience dictates the content, style and method of delivery. For each of these principles researchers need to observe the rules of communicating with specific groups. Effective transfer requires knowledge about how practitioners, decision makers, managers and policy makers function, whether the material can be mailed, published in scientific journals or delivered by hand (Bennett & Jessani, 2011).

At the same time the format in which the message is presented is important, such as the format of a journal article. Researchers follow the format the journal prescribes and, because of word limitations, have to reduce the message substantially. Still, the essence of the study needs to be conveyed to fellow researchers who want to see the findings, but will critically read the article, deciding whether the study used appropriate and rigorous methods. In the section following, the essence of the 1:3:25 principle is described and the basic rules highlighted.

The one-pager

The one-pager conveys clear and concise take-home messages for time-pressed decision makers and people who only have time to skim written material (Bennett & Jessani, 2011). This format increases the chance that it will actually be read and 'they also build capacity among researchers to express themselves with brevity' (Bennett & Jessani, 2011: 198).

The two-three-pager executive summary or policy brief

The executive summary (never more than three pages) should present the findings in a condensed manner to serve the needs of the busy decision maker. In this format the researcher would want to outline the issues that the researchers investigated, using plain and professional language, and present the facts in a logical manner. If possible, provide examples to the decision makers (in hospitals and the Department of Health, for example) which they can use and understand. It will also contain the bottom-line findings of the research. The executive summary differs from the academic abstract in the sense that it tells a story where the most important information is presented first and only subsequently followed by the background and context. This audience is not interested in the approach, methods and other technical details. The researcher can formulate that in one sentence if needs be. However, the researcher should focus on getting the essence of the research across as accurately as possible.

The aim of a two-three-pager is to frame a potential issue and / or problem, show possible solutions in context, and make specific recommendations. More specifically it can be developed using the following structure, as recommended by Bennett and Jessani (2011):

1. The length of a brief depends on the intended audience and the stage of the issue. The title is brief and grabs the reader's attention immediately. It also provides an overview of the problem, its

relevance, the reasons why action is necessary, and specific recommendations. This usually appears on the first page.

2. Statement of the problem: a good way to do this is to ask a question that requires a decision. Avoid 'Why' and focus instead on 'What', 'How', 'When', etc.

3. Background and/or context to the problem and its importance: the essential facts to convince an audience that the problem requires urgent attention and action.

4. Pre-existing policies: what has been done in the past when dealing with such a problem and/or what is in place now, if anything, to deal with the problem?

5. Policy options: suggest some alternative ways to address the problem.

6. The most important question to ask is to whom the brief should be given, and how is it to get onto that desk?

The 25-pager report

After the executive summary has convinced the decision maker to read the entire report, this format can be used to give more information about the research itself, still avoiding academic jargon. The report usually consists of the following important principles (Bennett & Jessani, 2011):

1. Context: the policy issue or managerial problem will be outlined here and the current state of the art and research.

2. Implications: the researcher states what his/her research means for the decision maker – the implications must be specific to the particular audience as there may be differences in what is important to different audiences.

3. Approach: a brief outline of the methods, the study design, data sources and details of the sample.

With what effect? Measuring the impact of knowledge transfer

Researchers need to account for each aspect of their research, and the same principle applies to knowledge transfer. The nature of the research and the message should guide the researcher as to the type of effect required. Raising awareness could be an outcome, but uptake into current practice or a change in behaviour and beliefs may be relevant outcomes. Ultimately informing policy development or change may be an outcome, or a combination of these outcomes.

The uptake of new research information can be observed in three forms of knowledge use. These three types of knowledge use are (1) instrumental use (knowledge is applied directly and specifically), (2) conceptual use (knowledge is used for general enlightenment); and (3) symbolic use (research is used to legitimise and sustain predetermined positions).

Evaluation of the impact of knowledge transfer is still a new field in which more work is required (Eccles, 2005). The complexity of healthcare systems, and their unique situations, experiences and needs, will influence health professionals' adoption and implementation decisions (Tsui *et al,* 2006). Lomas *et al* (1993) remind researchers that a healthcare professional is not an empty slate waiting for information and therefore one must understand the complexity of factors influencing the uptake of new research-based information.

Researchers are using a number of well-known instruments to measure the impact of knowledge transfer, such as Champion and Leach's Research Utilisation Questionnaire (Champion & Leach, 1989), the BARRIERS scale (Funk *et al,* 1991) and Lavis's assessment tool for measuring the clinical decision-making impact of applied research (Lavis *et al,* 2003). However, Lavis *et al* (2003) recommend that research needs to go beyond the 'use' of research findings to 'how' it is used.

Conclusion

Knowledge transfer is an inherent part of a research study. The process of knowledge transfer is complex, with little empirical evidence to guide researchers. Firstly, researchers use a multiplicity of terms to describe the process of knowledge transfer. Researchers must be upfront with their understanding of the concept and recognise that these definitions are often socially and politically motivated. Clarity on which terminology to use saves time and focuses a KT team's knowledge transfer plan.

Secondly, and because of the poor conceptualisation of knowledge transfer, there are no tried and tested theories that can be used to guide researchers. Using the metaphor from the work of Estabrooks *et al* (2006: 13) we conclude that 'theories provide maps for different kinds of terrain'. These kinds of terrain include the healthcare setting, researchers and research users (administrators, regulators, patients and advocacy groups). Healthcare settings are complex environments and researchers and research users need to face complex, multiple and competing demand forces when it comes to the implementation of new knowledge.

From the above it is clear that not only do we need multiple theories to guide our knowledge transfer plan, but it is also important that the researchers choose appropriate knowledge transfer strategies and products. Lastly, just as maps are terrain specific, knowledge transfer strategies should be context specific. A thorough understanding of the social characteristics of the research users and their organisational culture is needed to plan effectively for knowledge transfer. We have learned that a shared understanding of knowledge transfer should form part of the research proposal and implementation process to avoid spending valuable time in searching for an appropriate vocabulary.

Researchers not only need to know which of their research findings are important and need to be transferred, they also need to know their audiences to whom they want to transfer the findings. Appropriate formats to package the messages are needed based on a thorough understanding of their audiences. Unfortunately, research findings often do not reach research users in an understandable format. The most common way researchers transfer the findings of their research is by publication in peer-reviewed journals, which is often the strongest criterion for promotion. While conference presentations and posters come easier to researchers, writing one-pagers and policy briefs is difficult, especially as an in-depth understanding of the context and culture of the target audience is required. Communicating to the media is likewise a challenge to academia. Effective knowledge transfer thus needs appropriate training of researchers.

The trend is now towards including a complete end-of-grant knowledge transfer plan with a grant proposal. This plan needs to be clear as to the goals of the project's knowledge translation in terms of awareness raising and/or promotion of action. The goals of knowledge translation are determined by the research findings and may differ between audiences. It may therefore be the case that, once the audience is identified, the knowledge transfer strategy should be adapted to be appropriate for the audience. It also needs to be reviewed during the study.

We conclude by borrowing a quote from Bennett and Jessani (2011: 1):

> *Knowledge is like fine wine. The researcher brews it, the scientific paper bottles it, the peer review tastes it, the journal sticks a label on it, and archive systems store it carefully in a cellar. Splendid! Just one small problem: wine is only useful when somebody drinks it. Wine in a bottle does not quench thirst. Knowledge Translation (KT) opens the bottle, pours the wine into a glass, and serves it.*

References

Alberta Health Services - Alberta Mental Health Board. Alberta Mental Health Research Partnership Program (2009). *Knowledge Translation: A Synopsis of the Literature 2008*. Edmonton, Alberta: Harrington A, Beverley L, Barron G, Pazderka H, Bergerman L & Clelland S.

Alberta Addiction and Mental Health Research Partnership Program (2014). *Knowledge Translation Evaluation Planning Guide*. Edmonton, Alberta: Author.

Baumbusch J, Kirkham SR, Khan B, McDonald H, Semeniuck P & Tan E (2008). Pursuing common agendas: a collaborative model for knowledge translation between research and practice in clinical settings. *Res Nurs Health* 31: 130-140.

Bennett G & Jessani N (2011). *The Knowledge Translation Toolkit Bridging the Know-Do Gap: A Resource for Researchers*. International Development Research Centre (IDRC).

Canadian Institute of Health Research (CIHR) (2012). *Guide to Knowledge Translation Planning at CIHR: Integrated and End-of-Grant Approaches*. Ottawa, Ontario, Canada: CIHR.

Champion VL & Leach A (1989). Variables related to research utilization in nursing: an empirical investigation. *J Adv Nurs* 14: 705-710.

Cochrane LJ, Olson CA, Murray S, Dupuis M, Tooman T & Hayes S (2007). Gaps between knowing and doing: understanding and assessing the barriers to optimal health care. *J Contin Educ Health Prof* 27(2): 94-102.

Connor M & Norman P (1998). Health behaviour. In: Johnston DW & Johnston M (eds). *Health Psychology*. Oxford: Elsevier.

Duhamel F (2010). Implementing family nursing: how do we translate knowledge into clinical practice? Part II: The evolution of 20 years of teaching research and practice to a Center of Excellence in Family Nursing. *J Fam Nurs* 16: 8-25.

Eccles M, Grimshaw J, Walker A, Johnston M & Pitts N (2005). Changing the behavior of healthcare professionals: the use of theory in promoting the uptake of research findings. *J Clin Epidemiol* 58: 107-112.

Einarson A & Lockett D (2006). Do we have a knowledge transfer and translation plan at Teratogen Information Services? *Reprod Toxicol* 22: 542-545.

Estabrooks CA, Thompson DS, Lovely JR & Hofmeyer A (2006). A guide to knowledge translation theory. *J Contin Educ Health Prof* 26: 25-36.

Ferlie EB & Shortell SM (2001). Improving the quality of health care in the United Kingdom and the United States: a framework for change. *Milbank Q* 79: 281-315.

Funk SG, Champagne MT, Wiese RA & Tornquist EM. (1991). BARRIERS: the barriers to research utilization scale. *Appl Nurs Res* 4:39-45.

Goering P (2005). Knowledge transfer strategies for patient safety research: best practice and resources. Paper presented at Patient Safety and Quality Research conference in Canada.

Graham PJ (2008). *Knowledge Transfer in Theory and Practice: A Guide to the Literature*. Saskatoon, Canada: University of Saskatchewan.

Jacobson N, Butterill D & Goering P (2003). Development of a framework for knowledge translation: understanding user context. *J Health Serv Res Policy* 8(2): 94-99.

Lang ES, Wyer PS & Haynes RB (2007). Knowledge translation: closing the evidence-to-practice gap. *Ann Emerg Med* 49: 355-363.

Lave J & Wenger E (1991). *Situated Learning: Legitimate Peripheral Participation*. Cambridge, UK: Cambridge University Press.

Lavis JN, Robertson D, Woodside JM, McCleod CB, Abelson J (2003). How can research organisations more effectively transfer research knowledge to decision makers? *Millbank Q* 81(2): 221-248.

Lee RG & Garvin T (2003). Moving from information transfer to information exchange in health and health care. *Soc Sci Med* 56: 449-464.

Logan J & Graham ID (1998). Toward a comprehensive interdisciplinary model of health care research use. *Sci Comm 20*(2): 227-246.

Lomas J, Sisk JE, Stocking B (1993). From evidence to practice in the United States, the United Kingdom, and Canada. Milbank Quarterly 71(3):405-410.

Schuster M, McGlynn E, Brook RH (1998). How good is the quality of health care in the United States? *Millbank Q* 76: 563.

Straus SE, Green ML, Bell DS, Badgett R, Davis D, Gerrity M, Ortiz E, Shaneyfelt TM, Whelan C, Mangrulkar R and the Society of General Internal Medicine Evidence-Based Medicine Task Force (2004). Evaluating the teaching of evidence based medicine: conceptual framework. *BMJ* 329: 1029-1032 .

Tsui L, Chapman SA, Schnirer L & Steward S (2006). *A Handbook on Knowledge Sharing. Strategies and Recommendations for Researchers, Policymakers, and Service Providers*. Community University partnership for the Study of Children, Youth and Families. Alberta, Canada: University of Alberta.

Weiss CH (1979). The many meanings of research utilization. *Public Adm Rev* 39(6): 426-431.

Wenger E (1998). Communities of Practice: Learning, Meaning, and Identity. Cambridge UK: Cambridge University Press.

World Health Organization (2006). Bridging the "Know–Do" Gap – meeting on knowledge translation in global health 10-12 October 2005. Geneva, Switzerland: World Health Organization, Geneva, Switzerland. Available from: www.who.int/kms/WHO_EIP_KMS_2006_2.pdf

CHAPTER 6

A salutogenic perspective on maternity care for migrant women

Berit Viken, Marie-Clare Balaam and Anne Lyberg

Introduction

This chapter looks at migrant women and maternity care in Europe from a salutogenic perspective, drawing on the work of Aaron Antonovsky and other key scholars in the area of wellbeing and public health (Antonovsky, 1979; Antonovsky, 1987; Eriksson & Lindström, 2008). It considers the ways in which a salutogenic approach would deepen our understanding of the maternity needs and experiences of women who migrate to Europe. Using case studies from research work in Norway we assert that a salutogenic approach, while acknowledging the challenges faced by migrant women, would also recognise more fully the strengths, resilience and coping strategies of these women as they navigate pregnancy and motherhood in their new countries.

Migrants in Europe

The United Nations Department of Economic and Social Affairs (UNDESA) determined that worldwide in 2013 there were 232 million people living outside their country of origin (UNDESA, 2013). In Europe migrants make up an increasing part of the population in all 28 European Union (EU) states, which are popular reception countries for many migrants. During 2012, 1.7 million people migrated to the EU and a similar number of people migrated between EU states (Eurostat, 2015). The OECD has estimated that women comprise 48% of international migrants and, with the median age of migrants being between 29 and 43 years (this varies from region to region), many female migrants are of child-bearing age (OECD-UNDESA, 2013). The European Commission, considering the demographic future of Europe, noted that immigration can provide a valuable contribution to European nations in terms of positive demographic change as well as other economic, social and cultural benefits (Population Council, 2008). They emphasised, however, the need to create a family-friendly environment and to improve living conditions for families and children to allow all families to realise their aspirations. In light of these trends it is therefore crucial that those interested in providing optimal maternity care for women in Europe address the issue of the needs of migrant women.

In this chapter we will use the term migrant women to mean women who have moved from their country of origin to take up permanent residence in another country. However, we acknowledge that there are other definitions of the term migrant women used in different settings and that the use of different definitions, between countries, institutions and research communities, makes comparative analysis challenging (Rechel, Mladovsky, Devillé *et al*, 2011; Eurostat 2015; United Nations Educational, Scientific and Cultural Organisation (UNESCO), 2016; Statistics Norway, 2016).

The theory of salutogenesis

The salutogenic perspective used in this chapter draws on the work of sociologist Aaron Antonovsky and other researchers who have developed his ideas subsequently. Rather than taking a traditional medical approach focused on the roots of illness, Antonovsky coined the core concept of *salutogenesis* and posed the question 'What are the origins of health?' He explored the idea of health as a continuum from ease to dis-ease (Antonovsky, 1979). Antonovsky's answer to the question: 'What explains movements towards the health pole of the ease/dis-ease continuum?' was formulated in terms of a sense of coherence (SOC) and generalised resistance resources (GRR) (Lindström & Eriksson, 2010). In later work he assessed salutogenesis and the SOC in relation to other concepts, which sought to explain health and wellbeing in populations, including hardiness and resilience (Antonovsky, 1987; Kobasa, 1982; Werner & Smith, 1982; Lindström & Eriksson, 2010). Work on resilience focused on understanding the protective factors which act to maintain health and on how individuals survive in spite of adversity. This provided the basis for work which then focused on the promotion of health. Lindström and Eriksson have elaborated salutogenic theory using the metaphor 'Health in the River of Life' (Lindström & Eriksson, 2010). The theory of salutogenesis corresponds closely with the key principles in the Ottawa Charter for Health Promotion from WHO (WHO, 2010) and is useful in developing positive public health policies (Langeland & Vinje, 2013).

The SOC is the capability to perceive that one can manage in any situation independent of whatever else is happening in life. Three types of life experience shape an individual's SOC: consistency (comprehensibility), load balance (manageability) and participating in shaping outcomes (meaningfulness) (Antonovsky, 1987; Langeland &Vinje, 2013).

GRRs are biological, material and psychosocial factors that make it easier for people to perceive their lives as consistent, structured and understandable (Langeland &Vinje, 2013). Typical GRRs include: money, knowledge, experience, social support, culture, intelligence, tradition and ideologies. People with these kinds of resources available to them have a better chance of dealing positively with the challenges they may face in their lives. Migration can affect migrant women's GRRs both in a positive and negative way. Their living conditions, for example, may be better than in their country of origin but their social networks may be poorer.

It is important to explore issues such as, what is it that creates meaning in the lives of migrant women and helps them cope with their life in a new country as they give birth and raise their children? What are the conditions which affect their SOC, and how can they be understood in the light of ecological systems theory? (Bronfenbrenner, 1979).

Migrants' adaptation in a new cultural context

Riedel *et al* have proposed an integrative theoretical framework of acculturation and salutogenesis which provides a useful lens through which to view migrant experiences (Riedel *et al*, 2011). They consider the effect of resource factors on positive mental health outcomes in the migrant population. Their framework combines Berry's acculturation model, which illustrates the main factors that affect an individual's adaptation in a new country, and salutogenic theory (Berry, 2006a; Berry, 2006b). The four acculturative strategies used by immigrants are integration, assimilation, separation and marginalisation. Research on these strategies has revealed that integration is associated with the best psychological and sociocultural adaptation of an individual to life in their new country (Liebkind, 2002; Scottham & Dias, 2010; Sam & Berry, 2011). Riedel *et al* contend that it is essential to understand the context of resources, which can be psychological, social, institutional or cultural, in order to get an understanding of the psychological acculturation processes (Riedel *et al*, 2011). Resources and adequate strategies influence the outcome of coping processes and lead to variable degrees of adaptation. In a salutogenic perspective migration is an enduring and demanding change in one's life situation (Antonovsky, 1987).

The reproductive health of migrant women in Europe

The healthcare needs of migrant women have been an area of concern, both nationally and internationally, for academics, policy makers and international agencies, with a particular focus on issues of sexual and maternal health including access to maternal care and maternal and neonatal outcomes (International Organisation for Migration (IOM), 2009; Reeske & Razum, 2011; International Women's Health Coalition (IWHC), 2013; Médecins du Monde, 2014). Research suggests that many migrant women struggle to access optimal maternity care in Europe and commonly have worse maternal outcomes than native-born women (Essen, Hanson, Ostergren *et al*, 2000; Bollini, Pampallona, Wanner *et al*, 2009; Gissler, Alexander, Macfarlane, 2009; Balaam, Akerjordet, Lyberg *et al*, 2013).

This is due to a range of social, political and economic factors, which commonly intersect, during the period of migration and resettlement, to leave migrant women vulnerable to economic and social marginalisation. This in turn can affect their ability to maintain their mental and physical wellbeing in their new country of residence (Lyberg, Viken, Haruna *et al*, 2012; Haith-Cooper & Bradshaw, 2013). Many women struggle (in terms of salutogenic theory) to 'find meaning' and this is connected to unsuccessful communication and lack of connection with healthcare professionals, as they strive to cope and manage while struggling to achieve a safe pregnancy and birth and maintain a sense of bodily integrity (Balaam, Akerjordet, Lyberg *et al*, 2013).

It is, however, important to note the heterogeneous nature of migrant women and their experiences. The category 'migrant women' is a very broad one and includes women who have chosen to move for a range of economic or social reasons and those who have been subject to forced migration arriving in Europe as refugees, both documented and undocumented, asylum seekers or those who have been trafficked. Research reflecting this heterogeneity, suggests that some migrant women have maternal and newborn outcomes similar to native-born women. Others, notably refugees, asylum seekers, undocumented migrants and women from certain geographical regions, are much more vulnerable to receiving sub-optimal maternity care and having significantly worse outcomes than native populations (Lalchandani, Macquillan & Sheil, 2001; Gagnon, Zimbeck, Zeitlin *et al*, 2009; Lewis, 2007; Urquia, Glazier, Blondel *et al*, 2010; Platform for International Cooperation on Undocumented Migrants (PICUM), 2011).

Pathological and risk perspectives in maternity care research

Much research in maternity care focuses on the prevention of adversity rather than on the promotion of health (Smith, Daly, Lundgren *et al*, 2014; Perez-Botella, Downe, Meier Magistretti *et al*, 2014). In a recent review, Perez-Botella *et al* (2014) found that salutogenic theory is rarely used in maternity care research with healthy participants (Perez-Botella, Downe, Meier Magistretti *et al*, 2014). An increase in research that uses salutogenically focused outcomes could provide a balance to the current over-emphasis on pathology in maternity care design. This lack of a salutogenic approach is also evident in the majority of research work on migrant women. Most of the papers (published between 2000 and 2012) reviewed for Balaam *et al*'s paper on migrant women's experiences of maternity care used a pathological approach showing the deficiency of the care offered to women and focusing on negative outcomes (Balaam, Akerjordet, Lyberg *et al*, 2013). In contrast, it is possible to highlight ways in which, despite the very real obstacles faced by migrant women, many demonstrate resilience and agency and have positive experiences and outcomes against this background of challenge.

Another way of looking beyond a risk-based approach is to explore the specific factors which may explain the variations in neonatal and infant mortality rates and maternal outcomes for migrant women which, while tending to be higher than for the non-migratory population, are not uniformly so (IOM, 2009). Some migrant populations experience similar or better outcomes than the majority population, the so called 'healthy migrant effect', a term commonly explored in US research but less so in European research. Studies have explored the range of factors that may help to explain these differences including social and ethnic group, country of origin, refugee status, reception country policies, etc (Lalchandani, Macquillan & Sheil, 2001; Urquia, Glazier, Blondel *et al*, 2010; Rechel, Mladovsky, Devillé *et al*, 2011; Gagnon, DeBruyn, Essén *et al*, 2014; Gibson-Helm, Teede, Block *et al*, 2014). Research taking a more salutogenic approach would explore both the differences within and between migrant groups in different settings, as well as the full range of factors that may help explain why some of these women have positive outcomes despite the challenges many face.

A systems approach on health in migrant women

In a salutogenic perspective it is important to focus on the strengths and resources of migrant women in their social context, and to explore what makes migrant women move towards the 'ease' as opposed to the 'dis-ease' end of the health continuum. What are migrant women's capabilities to make good choices for their own health and wellbeing and for that of their babies and their families and how can their capabilities be strengthened? Hovden has conducted a study which sought to identify factors that influenced immigrant women's creation of their lives in a new context (Hovden, 2009). The aim was to explore the possibilities open to women and approach the health situation of immigrants from a salutogenic perspective. The women she interviewed were actively participating in a centre for health and dialogue (Primary Medical Workshop – PMV). The centre aims to improve the health and wellbeing of immigrant women in Oslo by seeking to empower women by focusing on their strengths and resources. This research identified the process of using one's resources, and experiencing mastery and a feeling of usefulness as the most important factors in influencing the development of these women's wellbeing in their new home country.

The integration of migrants into a new society depends on both personal and wider environmental factors. A nation's immigration policy establishes the nature of the environment in which the migrants have to live. The policy defines the legislative and bureaucratic structures within which they are located and affects their physical, social and economic integration into their new community. This sense of environment is also crucial when considering maternity care. Higginbottom *et al* compared migration and maternity care in Germany, Canada and the United Kingdom, and found that, while the design and delivery of maternal health services play a crucial role in ensuring positive experiences and good maternity outcomes for migrant women, these services must be understood within a much wider framework (Higginbottom, Reime, Bharj *et al*, 2013). Bronfenbrenner's *ecological model* provides a framework to study an individual's relationship within communities and society in general (Bronfenbrenner, 1979). The model was originally used to explain how a child's development is influenced by different environments, but is now considered to provide a valuable perspective in wider contexts. Bronfenbrenner identified four environmental systems with which an individual interacts: the *micro, meso, exo* and *macrosystem*. The *microsystem* refers to the institutions and groups that most directly influence the person's development, including: family, school, religious institutions, neighbourhood and peers. The migrant woman's life in a family and connections to other relatives and friends are part of the microsystem. The *mesosystem* involves relations between microsystems and connections between settings. Migrant women's interactions with individuals and institutions in the local community, such as the health services, make up the mesosystem. The *exosystem* involves links between a social setting in which the individual does not play an active role and her immediate context. Officials and administrators of the municipal and governmental institutions with whom women have no direct contact, but whose actions and policies still affect their lives, constitute the exosystem. The *macrosystem* describes the culture in which individuals live. The national authorities are part of the macrosystem.

In a review of qualitative studies, which focused on migrant women's perceptions of their needs and experiences related to maternity care, the authors contended that there is a relationship between their experiences of social inequality and access to pre, intra- and postpartum care (Balaam, Akerjordet & Lyberg, 2013). In the analysis there emerged one theme 'Preserving one's integrity in the new country' and two key aspects: 'Struggling to find meaning' and 'Caring relationships'. The results show that migrant women are in a vulnerable situation when pregnant and giving birth and that their access to health services must be improved to better meet their needs and allow them to build on their own strengths and resources. Caring relationships, support from healthcare professionals and members of primary support networks such as husbands, were important sources of strength. It is suggested that this vulnerability can be reduced by strengthening the continuity of care these women receive and by providing a caring relationship to help them find a sense of meaning in their new country (Balaam, Akerjordet & Lyberg, 2013).

In work considering the role of healthcare professionals in providing care for migrant women and focusing on the experiences of Norwegian healthcare professionals, Lyberg *et al* show that midwives and other health professionals encountered challenges in their interactions with migrant women in terms of managing and supporting educational, relational and cultural diversity (Lyberg & Severinsson, 2010). For example, providing continuity of care was sometimes difficult because some women did not always attend appointments, and women's varying educational and health informational needs, for example linked to birth control, also presented challenges. However, they found that, whilst migrant women often had different expectations of the content of maternity care than Norwegian women, they did expect to be treated with respect and care by skilful healthcare professionals.

Maternal health coping strategies – an example from Norway

A study from Norway has demonstrated that a sense of coherence (SOC) appears to influence migrant women's coping strategies when they become pregnant and give birth to a child (Viken, Lyberg & Severinsson, 2015). Women who participated in this study described how, even though their life was stressful, being pregnant and having a child gave them hope for the future. For these women the most meaningful task was taking care of their own and their baby´s health during pregnancy and childbirth. This is consistent with other studies, which highlight childbirth as a positive life event (Liamputtong & Naksook, 2003; Etowa, 2012).

Meaningfulness can be seen as the most important and motivational component in SOC (Antonovsky, 1979). When the women in the Norwegian study longed for their home country, they focused on safety for themselves and their children. Experiencing comfort and social security in a safe society constituted a major part of the women's meaningfulness. One participant said: *'Sometimes when I think of moving back, I remind myself of how safe our future is in Norway. I think it is a good environment for the children, with fresh air and clean, safe food'* (Viken, Lyberg & Severinsson, 2015).

The coping strategy of balancing their sense of belonging to family members and institutions in Norway with the sense of belonging that they felt to their relatives in their country of origin, also affected the women's sense of meaningfulness. Most of the women in the study maintained close links with family members in their country of origin through the internet, telephone and/or international travel. This can be considered part of the macrosystem and is supported by other studies that have a transnational perspective on migration. The identity and social practices of migrants transcend national borders, and migrants retain lasting ties with their country of origin (Levitt, 2001).

Alongside their links to their countries of origin women also found opportunities to create links to their new countries. For example, in order for newly arrived immigrants to be properly integrated, it is important that they can obtain work and an education and take part in society in other ways. In Norway the government runs the *Introductory Programme* which includes training in the Norwegian language and social studies for adult immigrants. The purpose of this programme is to increase the possibility of newly arrived immigrants participating in working and social life and to increase their financial independence. One participant who was asked about living in the municipality said: '*I am very positive to the municipality. I have got all the information I need about pregnancy and the delivery. I have also had the opportunity to learn Norwegian and earn money by going to the Introductory Programme*' (Viken, Lyberg & Severinsson, 2015).

The Introductory Programme is provided in the community and thus forms part of migrant women's mesosystem. In the mesosystem all interaction takes place across settings (Bronfenbrenner, 1979). Active participation in a new setting can increase the women's capabilities, for example, language skills can help them to comprehend health information and social structures in Norwegian society. Participation also strengthens social networks and makes daily life more manageable by creating independence through not having to rely on translation by family members and interpreters. The ability to communicate in Norwegian also provides a stronger sense of belonging to society as it enables the women to strengthen their social networks and start new activities such as entering into paid employment. Nussbaum contends that economic independence enhances women's self-respect and capacity for choice (Nussbaum, 2011). Seeking information and support from family and healthcare professionals is a coping strategy where migrant women interact both within their microsystem and with the maternal and child health services, which are a part of their mesosystem. Information and support in pregnancy increases women's comprehensibility and manageability.

The maternal health coping strategies of migrant women are also influenced by their health literacy, a composite term used to describe the capacities of persons to meet the complex demands related to health information in modern society (Nutbeam, 2010). It is a resource that equips people to navigate healthcare systems, critically assess information and take greater control of their health. Health literacy applies to the development of skills and capacities that enable migrant women to exert greater control over their health and the factors that shape it. Consequently, health literacy affects women's maternal health coping strategies.

Language courses, maternal and child health services as well as social media interactions all contribute to migrant women's health literacy and thus their sense of comprehensibility and manageability. Migrant women's comprehensibility also involves their original cultural traditions and formal education. Some of the participants in the Norwegian study had low levels of formal education, which affected their health literacy. The women who could not read and write were largely dependent on verbal information from healthcare professionals to increase their comprehensibility. Consistent with these findings is the need for more innovative forms of communication that go beyond the written word (Higginbottom, Bell & Arsenault, 2012). In their encounters with healthcare professionals the women who did not speak Norwegian were highly dependent on interpreters to achieve understanding. The reliance on interpreters and translated material can add complexities to these interactions due to challenges in the procedures and the differences in the meaning of concepts between languages and cultures (Liamputtong, 2010).

Consequences for maternity care

The link between social conditions and health has been an area of research and public policy for several decades. This work has demonstrated that the more favoured people are, socially and economically, the better their health (Marmot Review, 2010; Phelan, Link & Tehranifar, 2010; WHO, 2010; Royal College of Nursing, 2012). Working to reduce social inequalities within health means making positive efforts to ensure that all social groups achieve the same levels of health and life expectancy. Migrants can be comparatively healthy, but they often face particular health challenges (Rechel, Mladovsky, Devillé *et al*, 2011). These are often due to their experience of poorer social and economic conditions (Healthcare Commission, 2008; Raleigh, Hussey, Seccombe *et al*, 2010; Eurohealth, 2014) as well as issues relating to difficulties in accessing appropriate healthcare (Bischoff, Bovier, Isah *et al*, 2003; Novak-Zezula, Schulze, Karl-Trummer *et al*, 2005; Gagnon, DeBruyn, Essén *et al*, 2014). This can be connected to the fact that the health needs of migrants are often poorly understood, communication with healthcare providers is inadequate and health systems are not prepared to respond adequately.

The aim of health promotion is to achieve equity in health. Reorienting health services is an important strategy in the Ottawa Charter for Health Promotion and implies that the health sector should move in a health promotion direction, beyond its responsibility for providing clinical and curative services (WHO, 1986). It is vital that this leads to a change of attitude towards the organisation of health services, with the focus being on the total needs of the individual as a whole person and her or his wellbeing in the widest sense.

Pursuing a salutogenic approach to maternity care and research about migrant women would encourage healthcare professionals, policy makers and maternity service users to consider maternity care from a health-oriented and person-centred perspective as opposed to one based on morbidity and mortality. The provision and organisation of maternity care should be adjusted to the needs of all migrant women, taking account of the range of factors that can affect access to healthcare in order to ensure that these women can access the same quality of care as native-born women (Gagnon, DeBruyn, Essén *et al*, 2014). In order to provide culturally competent care, healthcare professionals must be culturally sensitive and aware of their own cultural heritage (Leininger, 2001; Ramsden, 2002; Seeleman, Suurmond & Stronks, 2009). To gain a better cultural sensitivity, healthcare leaders should acknowledge the need for clinical supervision in practice, especially for healthcare professionals working with migrants. Clinical supervision and leadership are necessary for professional development and the acquisition of new skills, which involve reflection on practice. Midwives interviewed in a study by Lyberg *et al* appreciated being given the opportunity to reflect on their practice with their colleagues (Lyberg, Viken, Haruna *et al*, 2012). Another study contended that midwives' supervisory styles were related to their ability to create a trusting and caring relationship, to demonstrate problem-solving capacities and to show willingness, preparedness and courage to support pregnant women (Liamputtong & Naksook, 2013). Co-operation with other sectors and multidisciplinary work is part of a salutogenic approach and can strengthen migrant women's capabilities and affect their wellbeing.

The salutogenic perspective in research on maternity care has been highlighted in the COST Action IS0907 'Childbirth Cultures, Concerns and Consequences: Creating a Dynamic Framework for Optimal Maternity Care' (Smith, Daly, Lundgren *et al*, 2014; Perez-Botella, Downe, Meier Magistretti *et al*, 2014). We advocate that a salutogenic perspective is especially appropriate for migrant women in order to build on their resources and strengths. For migrant women it is important to obtain a caring relationship with the midwife and feel secure. The sense of security is in turn dependent on the (cultural) competence and leadership of each individual midwife (Liamputtong & Naksook, 2003). Supervision and leadership have an impact on the quality of maternity care. In order to ensure continuity and a trusting relationship it is necessary to organise leadership and adopt flexible models that support migrant women's health.

References

Antonovsky A (1979). *Health, Stress and Coping*. San Francisco & London: Jossey-Bass Inc. Publishers.

Antonovsky A (1987). *Unraveling the Mystery of Health: How People Manage Stress and Stay Well*. London: Jossey-Bass Ltd.

Balaam M-C, Akerjordet K, Lyberg A, Kaiser B, Schoening E, Fredriksen A-M, Ensel A, Gouni O & Severinsson E (2013). A qualitative review of migrant women´s perceptions of their needs and experiences related to pregnancy and childbirth. *J Adv Nurs* 69 (9):1919-1930.

Berry JW (2006a). Acculturative stress. In: Wong PTP & Wong LCJ (eds). *Handbook of Multicultural Perspectives on Stress and Coping*. Dallas, Texas: Spring, pp287-298.

Berry JW (2006b). Stress perspectives on acculturation. In: Sam DL & Berry JW (eds). *The Cambridge Handbook of Acculturation Psychology*. New York: Cambridge University Press, pp43-57.

Bischoff A, Bovier PA, Isah R, Francoise G, Ariel E, Louis L (2003). Language barriers between nurses and asylum seekers: Their impact on symptom reporting and referral. *Soc Sci Med* 57(3): 503-512.

Bollini P, Pampallona S, Wanner, P, Kupelnick B (2009). Pregnancy outcome of migrant women and integration policy: a systematic review of the international literature. *Soc Sci Med* 68: 425-461.

Bronfenbrenner U (1979). *The Ecology of Human Development: Experiments by Nature and Design*. Cambridge, Massachusetts: Harvard University Press.

Eriksson M, Lindström B (2008). A salutogenic interpretation of the Ottawa Charter. *Health Promot Int* 23(2):190-199.

Essen B, Hanson BS, Ostergren P, Lindquist P, Gudmundsson S (2000). Increased perinatal mortality among sub-Saharan immigrants in a city-population in Sweden. *Acta Obstet Gynecol Scand* 79: 737-743.

Etowa JB (2012). Becoming a mother: the meaning of childbirth for African-Canadian women. *Contemp Nurse* 2012; 41:128-40

Eurohealth (2014). *Migrants and Health. Quarterly of the European Observatory on Health Systems and Policies* 20 (4). Available from: www.lse.ac.uk/LSEHealthAndSocialCare/pdf/eurohealth/VOL20No4/EH20.4-WEB-Version-16Dec14.pdf

Eurostat (2015). Population data. Available from: http://ec.europa.eu/eurostat/web/population-demography-migration-projections/population-data

Gagnon AJ, Zimbeck M, Zeitlin J, Alexander S, Blondel B, Buitendijk S, Desmeules M, Di Lallo D, Gagnon A, Gissler M, Glazier R, Heaman M, Korfker D, Macfarlane A, Ng E, Roth C, Small R, Stewart D, Stray-Pederson B, Urquia M & Vangen S (2009). Migration to western industrialised countries and perinatal health: a systematic review. *Soc Sci Med* 69(6): 934-946.

Gagnon A J, DeBruyn R, Essén B, Gissler M, Heaman M, Jeambey Z, Korfker D, McCourt C, Roth C, Zeitlin J, Small R for the ROAM Collaboration (2014). Development of the Migrant Friendly Maternity Care Questionnaire (MFMCQ) for migrants to Western societies: an international Delphi consensus process. *BMC Pregnancy Childbirth* 14: 200. Available from: www.biomedcentral.com/1471-2393/14/200

Gibson-Helm M, Teede H, Block A, Knight M, East C, Wallace EM & Boyle J (2014). Maternal health and pregnancy outcomes among women of refugee background from African countries: a retrospective, observational study in Australia. *BMC Pregnancy Childbirth* 14: 392.

Gissler M, Alexander S, Macfarlane A, Small R, Stray-Pedersen B, Zeitlin J, Zimbeck M, Gagnon A (2009). Stillbirths and infant deaths among migrants in industrialized countries. *Acta Obstet Gynecol Scand* 88(2): 134-148.

Haith-Cooper M, Bradshaw G (2013). Meeting the health and social needs of pregnant asylum seekers; midwifery students' perspectives. Part 3; the pregnant women within the global context; an inclusive model for midwifery education to address the needs of recently arrived migrant women in the UK. *Nurse Educ Today* 9: 1008-1013.

Healthcare Commission (2008). *Towards Better Births: A Review of Maternity Services in England.* Health Care Commission, London. 2008. Available from: http://webarchive.nationalarchives.gov.uk/20101014074803/http:/www.cqc.org.uk/_db/_documents/Towards_better_births_200807221338.pdf

Higginbottom G, Bell AS, Arsenault J & Pilay J (2012). An integrative review of experiences of maternity services for immigrant women in Canada. *Diversity and Equality in Health and Care* 9: 1-14.

Higginbottom GMA, Reime B, Bharj K, Chowbey P, Ertan K, Foster-Boucher C, Friedrich J, Gerrish K, Kentenich H, Mumtaz Z, O´Brien B & Salway S (2013). Migration and maternity: insights of context, health policy, and research evidence on experiences and outcomes from a three country preliminary study across Germany, Canada and the United Kingdom. *Health Care Women Int* 34(11): 936-965.

Hovden SL (2009). Exploring possibilities: a salutogenic perspective on health among immigrant women in Oslo. Master's thesis, Master of Philosophy in Health Promotion. University of Bergen.

International Organisation for Migration (IOM) (2009). *Maternal & Child Healthcare for Immigrant Populations.* Available from: www.migrant-health-europe.org/files/Maternal%20and%20Child%20Care_Background%20Paper%281%29.pdf

International Women's Health Coalition (2013). UN resolution calls on governments to provide sexual and reproductive health services to migrants. Available from: http://iwhc.org/press-release/un-resolution-calls-governments-provide-sexual-reproductive-health-services-migrants

Kobasa S (1982). The hardy personality: toward a social psychology of stress and health. In: Sanders G & Suls J (eds.) *Social Psychology of Health and Illness.* New Jersey: Lawrence Erlbaum Associates, pp3-32.

Lalchandani S, Macquillan K, Sheil O (2001). Obstetric profiles and pregnancy outcomes of immigrant women with refugee status. *Irish Med J* 94: 79-80.

Langeland E, Vinje HF (2013). The significance of salutogenesis and well-being in mental health promotion: from theory to practice. In: Corey L & Keyes M (eds). *Mental Well-Being: International Contributions to the Study of Positive Mental Health.* New York: Springer, pp299-329.

Leininger M (2001). *Cultural Care Diversity and Universality: A Theory of Nursing.* Sudbury, Massachusetts: Jones and Bartlett.

Levitt P (2001). *The Transnational Villagers.* Berkeley: University of California Press.

Lewis G (2007). *Confidential Enquiry into Maternal and Child Health Saving Mothers Lives: Reviewing Maternal Deaths to Make Motherhood Safer 2003-2005.* The seventh report on confidential enquiries into maternal deaths in the United Kingdom. London: CEMACH.

Liamputtong P & Naksook C (2003). Life as mothers in a new land: the experience of motherhood among Thai women in Australia. *Health Care Women Int* 24:650-668.

Liamputtong P (2010). *Performing Qualitative Cross-Cultural Research.* Cambridge: Cambridge University Press.

Liebkind K (2002). Acculturation. In: Brown R & Gaertner S (eds). *Blackwell Handbook of Social Psychology: Intergroup Processes.* Oxford: Blackwell, pp368-406.

Lindström B & Eriksson M (2010). *The Hitchhikers' Guide to Salutogenesis: Salutogenic Pathways to Health Promotion*. Folkhälsan: IUHP.

Lindström B & Eriksson M (2010). A salutogenic approach to tackling health inequalities. In: Morgan A, Davies M & Ziglio E (eds). *Health Assets in a Global Context: Theory, Methods, Action.* New York: Springer, pp17-40.

Lyberg A & Severinsson E (2010). Midwives' supervisory styles and leadership roles as experienced by Norwegian mothers in the context of fear of childbirth. *J Nurs Manag* 18(4): 391-399.

Lyberg A, Viken B, Haruna M & Severinsson E (2012). Diversity and challenges in Maternity care for migrant women. *J Nurs Manag* 20(2): 287-295.

Marmot Review (2010). *Fair Society, Healthy Lives.* The Marmot Review. Executive Summary. Strategic Review of Health Inequalities in England post-2010. Available from: www.ucl.ac.uk/marmotreview

Médecins du Monde (2014). *Access to Healthcare for the Most Vulnerable in a Europe in Social Crisis.* Available from: http://epha.org/medecins-du-monde-new-mdm-report-on-access-to-healthcare-for-the-most-vulnerable-in-a-europe-in-social-crisis-focus-on-pregnant-women-and-children

Novak-Zezula S, Schulze B, Karl-Trummer U, Krajic K & Pelikan JM (2005). Improving interpreting in clinical communication: models of feasible practice from the European project 'Migrant-friendly Hospitals'. *Diversity Health Soc Care* 2(3):223-232.

Nussbaum M (2011). *Creating Capabilities: The Human Development Approach.* Harvard University Press.

Nutbeam D (2010). The evolving concept of health literacy. *Soc Sci Med* 67: 2072-2078.

Organisation for Economic Co-operation and Development – United Nations Department of Economic and Social Affairs (OECD-UNDESA) (2013). *World Migration in Figures.* Available from: www.oecd.org/els/mig/World-Migration-in-Figures.pdf

Perez-Botella M, Downe S, Meier Magistretti C, Lindstrom B & Berg M (2014). The use of salutogenesis theory in empirical studies of maternity care for healthy mothers and babies. *Sex Reprod Healthc* 6(1): 33-39.

Phelan JC, Link BG & Tehranifar P (2010). Social conditions as fundamental causes of health inequalities: theory, evidence and policy implications. *J Health Soc Behav* 51: S28.

Platform for International Cooperation on Undocumented Migrants (PICUM) (2011). *Preventing Undocumented Pregnant Women and Children from Accessing Health Care: Fostering Health Inequalities in Europe.* Available from: http://picum.org/en/publications/conference-and-workshop-reports/25872

Population Council (2008). The European Parliament on the demographic future of Europe. *Population and Development Review* 34(2): 381-386. www.jstor.org/stable/25434698

Raleigh VS, Hussey D, Seccombe I & Hallt K (2010). Ethnic and social inequalities in women's experience of maternity care in England: results of a national survey. *J Res Soc Med* 103(5): 188-198.

Ramsden I (2002). Teaching cultural safety. *N Z Nurs J* 85(5): 21-23.

Rechel B, Mladovsky P, Devillé W, Rijks B, Roumyana P-B & McKee M (2011). *Migration and Health in the European Union.* European Observatory on Health Systems and Policies Series, 2011. Available from: www.euro.who.int/__data/assets/pdf_file/0019/161560/e96458.pdf

Reeske A & Razum O (2011). Maternal and child health – from conception to first birthday. In: Rechel B, Mladovsky P, Devillé W, Rijks B, Roumyana P-B & McKee M (eds). *Migration and Health in the European Union.* European Observatory on Health Systems and Policies Series. Open University Press.

Riedel J, Wiesmann U & Hannich H-J (2011). An integrative theoretical framework of acculturation and salutogenesis. *Int Rev Psychiatry* 23(6): 555-654.

Royal College of Nursing (RCN) (2012). *Health inequalities and the social determinants of health*. Available from: www.rcn.org.uk/about-us/policy-briefings/pol-0112

Sam DL & Berry JW (2011). *The Cambridge Handbook of Acculturation Psychology*. New York: Cambridge University Press.

Scottham KM & Dias RH (2010). Acculturative strategies and the psychological adaptation of Brazilian migrants to Japan. *Identity* 10: 284-303.

Seeleman C, Suurmond J & Stronks K (2009). Cultural competence: a conceptual framework for teaching and learning. *Med Educ* 43: 229-237.

Smith V, Daly D, Lundgren I, Eri T, Benstoem C & Devane D (2014). Salutogenically focused outcomes in systematic reviews of intrapartum interventions: a systematic review of reviews. *Midwifery* 30(4):151-156.

Statistics Norway (2016). Norway: http://ssb.no

United Nations Department of Economic and Social Affairs (UN-DESA) (2013). Number of international migrants rises above 232 million. Available from: www.un.org/en/development/desa/news/population/number-of-international-migrants-rises.html

United Nations Educational, Scientific and Cultural Organisation (UNESCO) (2016). Definition of migrant. Available from: www.unesco.org/new/en/social-and-human-sciences/themes/international-migration/glossary/migrant

Urquia ML, Glazier RH, Blondel B, Zeitlin J, Gissler M, Macfarlane A, Ng E, Heaman M, Stray-Pedersen B & Gagnon AJ (2010). International migration and adverse birth outcomes: role of ethnicity, region of origin and destination. *J Epidemiol Community Health* 64(3): 243-251.

Viken B, Lyberg A & Severinsson E (2015). Maternal health coping strategies of migrant women in Norway. *Nursing Res Prac.* Epub Mar 17: 878040.

Werner E & Smith R (1982). *Vulnerable but Invincible: A Longitudinal Study of Resilient Children and Youth*. New York: McGraw Hill.

World Health Organization (WHO) (1986). The Ottawa Charter for Health Promotion. Available from: www.who.int/healthpromotion/conferences/previous/ottawa

World Health Organization (WHO) (2010). What are social determinants of health? Available from: www.who.int/social_determinants/sdh_definition

CHAPTER 7

Migrant midwives: contributing to a different culture

Sarah Church and Olga Gouni

Introduction

Within contemporary society, the growth in global healthcare services has increased the demand for healthcare professionals (Clark *et al*, 2006). However, the movement of health professionals is currently provoking a global health workforce crisis in which the loss of skilled health professionals from low to medium income countries to high-income countries places a further burden on health systems which are already under resourced. The World Health Organization (WHO) (WHO, 2006: 101) state that: 'when a country has a fragile health system, the loss of its workforce can bring the whole system close to collapse and the consequences can be measured in lives lost'. Whilst the report identified that 57 countries have critical shortages equivalent to a global deficit of 2.4 million doctors, nurses and midwives, the greatest shortfall is seen in sub-Saharan Africa and south-east Asia. For example, data compiled by the WHO (2006) indicate that 5% (28,597) of nurses and midwives trained in sub-Saharan Africa work in Organisation for Economic Co-operation and Development (OECD) countries such as Canada, Denmark, Finland, Ireland, Portugal, the United Kingdom (UK) and the United States of America (USA). Examples include 34% (3,183) from Zimbabwe; 13% (2,267) from Ghana; 18% (2,000) from Lesotho and 18% (781) from Mauritius. This outflow or 'brain drain' of health-skilled professionals from developing countries aggravates an already desperate situation resulting in more stress for the health professionals who remain. Moreover, some studies suggest that the migration of healthcare professionals from sub-Saharan Africa, for example, has negative effects on the provision and quality of care in the countries which they have left (Mills *et al*, 2011).

As a result of growing workforce concerns and the worsening health issues within these countries, the Global Health Workforce Alliance and the Health Workforce Department of the WHO have launched a new project entitled 'Brain drain to brain gain' with the main objective of improving the management of the migration of healthcare professionals from sub-Saharan Africa and Asian countries. Furthermore, a global code of practice on international recruitment was developed (WHO, 2010) to address the ethical issues created by the movement of health professionals and as a means of protecting the health systems within developing countries. Similar codes for international recruitment have since been developed by OECD countries; for example, the UK, Canada and Norway, which underpin recruitment policies and practices.

However, the migration of healthcare professionals cannot be seen in isolation and must be considered in relation to social, political and economic contexts. The World Health Organization (WHO, 2006) states that healthcare workers are experiencing increasing stress and insecurity due to complex challenges within health systems driven by demographic, epidemiological and political changes, such as financing health provision, which lead to human rights violations. As a result, healthcare workers seek opportunities in dynamic and well-resourced environments which provide more job satisfaction and job security. In contrast, reports of the underutilisation of skilled health professionals are also evident in many developing countries. A lack of opportunity to work creates further discontent. WHO emphasise that 'Poverty, imperfect private labour markets, lack of public funds, bureaucratic red tape and political interference produce this paradox of shortages in the midst of underutilized talent' (WHO, 2006: p xviii).

Against this global concern, changes to European law support the free movement of workers across Europe creating further opportunities for mobility. More specifically, professional mobility is one of the 'four freedoms' of the EU which act as the cornerstone of the European framework. This change has led to the active recruitment of health professionals by National Health Service (NHS) employers faced with increased shortages in the nursing and midwifery workforce. This activity has raised further concerns about the balance of health systems and its performance to meet the healthcare needs of different populations across the European Union (EU) (Palm *et al*, 2011).

Recent European workforce studies, namely Mobility of Health Professionals (MoHprof) (Tjadens *et al*, 2013) and the Health Professional Mobility in the European Union study (PROMeTHEUS) (Wismar *et al*, 2011), have attempted to address questions in relation to the magnitude and impact of mobility across European countries. However, the focus of these studies is largely placed on doctors, nurses and dentists, with only a brief consideration of midwives. Against this background, this chapter will explore the issue of migration in relation to midwives. A broad approach is taken due to limited literature, to consider migration in the context of registration and competency assessment. The process and experience of acculturation will be examined by the application of a salutogenic model and will consider the wider issues of workforce integration. This chapter will conclude with a focus on the development of the global midwife and considers some of the challenges and opportunities for this role. Recommendations for further research will be offered.

Midwives and migration

Patterns of migration associated with healthcare professionals are understood in terms of migration between developing countries, migration from developing countries to developed countries, and migration between developed countries. However, the mobility of midwives has received little attention within the literature in comparison to other healthcare professionals such as nurses (Bourgeault *et al*, 2011). Whilst midwives are known to have a history of migration, there is limited research on the extent of migration, mobility patterns and the experiences of midwives. One explanation for this is the incomplete data on the mobility of midwives. Registration data for midwives are generally combined with data on nurses. Therefore, as Bourgeault *et al* (2011) suggest, any discussion of midwives is considered within the context of nurse migration. This is further supported by Sidebotham and Ahern (2011) who suggest:

> *It remains difficult, however, to identify issues specific to the midwifery profession as most of the literature examining the global movement of healthcare professionals includes midwifery as a sub branch of nursing.*

Against this background, the relationship between migration and the global shortage of midwives is noted in relation to sub-Saharan Africa, where maternal deaths are the highest in the world. Whilst the numbers of midwives represented across countries at greatest risk are difficult to ascertain, reasons for the migration of midwives from sub-Saharan Africa have been described as difficult working conditions underpinned by poor resources, high workload and poor pay, together with the threat and incidences of violence and concerns for personal safety. Poor education and training opportunities and facilities are also evident for specialist midwives.

Our current understanding of the mobility of midwives relies on data derived from specific countries which, in the absence of extensive literature, provide some insights into possible patterns between particular countries.

Countries within mainland Europe and Scandinavian countries have their own history of receiving healthcare professionals, influenced by cross-border relationships and linguistic capabilities. For example, Spain receives healthcare professionals from Latin America, and Norway receives healthcare professionals from Sweden and Finland. The UK's colonial history has resulted in the migration of midwives from other English-speaking countries such as South Africa, Australia and the Caribbean. More recently the UK has received midwives from across Europe including Poland, Bulgaria, Italy and Spain (Church & Grey, 2012). A pan-London approach to fill vacant midwifery posts resulted in the recruitment of midwives from Belgium and Italy (Dunkley & Haider, 2011). In addition, midwives from the UK continue to travel the world using their midwifery qualifications to secure employment in countries such as Australia (Sidebotham & Ahern, 2011), New Zealand (Davies *et al,* 2010) and the Far East (Nursing and Midwifery Council (NMC), 2009).

Data from SEMMA (Sillogos, Epistimonon, Maion, Maieuton, Athinon) (a direct English translation is Association of Scientists - Midwives (Male & Female) of Athens, which is the official body of the Midwives Association of Athens) and the International Confederation of Midwives (ICM) indicate the number of midwives registered to work in Greece. In 2014 registration data revealed that there were 210 migrant midwives registered to work. Midwives were mainly from the ex-Soviet Union, Bulgaria, Poland and the Czech Republic. A small number of midwives came from the UK, Germany, Switzerland, France, South Africa, Peru and Uganda. A larger number of midwives came from Albania and many completed their midwifery studies in the Greek Midwifery Education system (Lymperi, 2014).

Knowledge of cross-border practices and political agreements provides some insights into the mobility of midwives. Offermanns *et al* (2011), in a case study of midwives moving from and to Austria, provide data in relation to the mobility of midwives. They note that, whilst its proximity to Germany enables more German midwives to work in Austria, data for newly registered midwives in 2008 indicate that Austria received 20 midwives from a number of countries including Bulgaria (n=2); France (n=1); the Islamic Republic of Iran (n=2); Italy (n=1); Poland (n=2); Turkey (n=1) and Germany (n=11). Data for all 322 practising midwives in Austria for 2008 include three categories: midwives with foreign citizenship (n=193); midwives categorised as foreign-born with Austrian citizenship (n=120); and Austrian-born, foreign-trained midwives (n=9). Of the 193 midwives with foreign citizenship, the largest number of midwives came from Germany (83); Poland (31); the Czech Republic (15) and Slovakia (12), whilst the remaining 52 midwives came from countries across Europe with one midwife from Chile. Of the foreign-born midwives with Austrian citizenship (n=120) the largest number of midwives came from the Philippines (n=30), Poland (n=30) and Germany (n=11). The outflow of midwives from Austria recorded for the same year included those who had applied for educational verification to work in other EU member states (n=5): Germany (n=1); Italy (n=1) with the remaining three midwives applying for visas to work in Australia (n=1), New Zealand (n=1) and the United Republic of Tanzania (n=1). This information presents a useful platform for the discussion of wider issues related to the process of registration for practice in other countries.

Registration and competency assessment

The impact of the mobility of midwives can be considered in relation to concerns about language ability, literacy skills and clinical competence of migrant midwives. This has led to revisions to the EU Directive on the Recognition of Professional Qualifications (Directive 2005/36/EC), in which additional language controls have been introduced (Department of Health, 2015). A focus on limiting risk to the public and the identification of who is 'fit to practise' are major considerations for regulators and for employers. Using the UK as an example of a country which is considered as a major destination for migrant healthcare professionals, the process of seeking registration to practise, either as a midwife from within the European Union (EU) and European Economic Area (EEA) (NMC, 2011) or from outside the EU/EEA, merits consideration. Since October 2014 the Nursing and Midwifery Council (NMC) has offered the Test of Competence for midwives who trained outside the EU/EEA who wish to register to work as a midwife in the UK (NMC, 2014). This includes a computer-based test of theoretical practice-based knowledge undertaken in test centres around the world, together with an objective-structured clinical examination (OSCE) completed in the UK. The opportunity for registration is also available for midwives who are refugees and asylum seekers, although specific guidance on registration is given to each midwife on an individual basis depending on availability of evidence.

For midwives who trained within the EU/EEA each midwife is assessed against the requirements for automatic recognition and acquired rights as set out in Directive 2005/36/EC. For automatic registration, qualifications gained from countries that joined the EU after 23 January 1983 will be assessed against standards set out in the directive. Others who completed their training before their countries joined the EU will be required to comply with acquired rights, which set out specific requirements for practice. Each midwife's qualifications and experiences are assessed. If automatic registration is not appropriate, the NMC advise the midwife on the most appropriate options (NMC, 2011).

Successful professional registration facilitates the migration of midwives but is dependent on the process of verification of qualifications and experience by the host country and is subject to co-operation and agreement between countries. In addition, the structure, composition and standards of midwifery education programmes are fundamental to the eligibility of midwives to work in other countries. Whilst countries do differ, broad requirements are set out in Directive 2005/36/EC to enable midwives to be assessed for registration elsewhere (http://ec.europa.eu/growth/single-market/services/qualifications/policy-developments/legislation/index_en.htm). For example, the registration process, SEMA-INC (Greece) follows European Guideline 36/2005 in which evidence of qualifications (translated into Greek), a passport and proficient Greek language skills are required before registration is approved. This equally applies to midwives from EU countries. For midwives from non-EU countries, a degree recognition is required (issued by ΔΟΑΤΑΠ), a residence and work permit and a Bilateral Agreement Certificate from the Ministry of Foreign Affairs. In addition, a transcript of training may be requested by the Board. Where a decision to approve registration is difficult, the midwife is required to contact the Professional Qualifications Recognition Council (ΣΑΕΠ) to make a decision regarding her application for registration.

A positive approach to the facilitation of a more coherent system was introduced by the formation of the Network of European Midwifery Regulators (NEMIR) in 2009. This is a joint initiative between the French Chamber of Midwives (L'Ordre des sages-femmes) and the Nursing and Midwifery Council (NMC). Whilst this network was established on an informal basis, the broad aim of the network is 'to improve the mutual understanding and exchange of best practices between regulators and competent authorities and to co-ordinate joint communications with EU decision makers on issues of mutual concern, especially in regard to EU legislation' (NEMIR, 2009). This network is made up of midwifery regulators and competent authorities representing 25 countries.

The Network of European Midwifery Regulators (NEMIR) has been welcomed as a means to address issues of fitness to practise and as a means to assess safety and risk. The emphasis on ensuring that registration procedures safeguard the safety of mothers and babies is paramount. Revisions to Directive 2005/36/EC stipulate that regulators should be proactive in the use of a warning system which will prevent 'rogue' professionals from moving across EU countries. Since its formation, the NEMIR has conducted two surveys on various issues including training and education requirements, and mobility issues. The most recent report also included a discussion of regulation and disciplinary procedures (NEMIR, 2009; NEMIR, 2010).

In the most recent report (NEMIR, 2010), the annual numbers of new registrants who qualified between 2003-2008 in other EU/EEA countries represent the movement of midwives across certain countries. Data for nine countries included in the report are represented in Table 1. These data indicate the existence of movement rather than a detailed picture of mobility. It could be concluded that Ireland, Norway, France and the UK have received larger numbers of midwives during these years compared to the other countries. It is understood that Ireland receives a large number of midwives from the UK, but further analysis would enable a more precise account of mobility patterns across these countries, including the source countries.

Table 1:

Annual number of new registrants qualified in a range of EU/EEA countries (excluding nationally qualified)

	2003	2004	2005	2006	2007	2008
Hungary (HU)	8	2	6	1	3	-
Cyprus (CY)	3	7	17	9	4	19
Austria (AT)	7	34	26	34	16	27
Ireland (IE)	53	46	51	110	133	100
Luxembourg (LU)	6	10	13	9	9	15
Norway (NO)	102	82	94	122	99	108
France (FR)	-	65	82	153	122	100
Portugal (PT)	-	2	4	6	0	1
United Kingdom (UK)	30	74	141	122	84	97

Source: Survey of European Midwifery Regulators 2010 (NEMIR, 2010)

The experience of acculturation

Ea *et al* (2008: 47) define acculturation as:

> *... a complex, multidimensional, and bidirectional process that involves the adopting of the behaviours and attitudes of the host country and relinquishing the behaviours and attitudes of the original culture.*

Much of the migration literature critically explores acculturation as cultural change encompassing the interrelation between concepts such as integration, assimilation and marginalisation, in which a focus is placed on the complexity of relationships between cultural groups at a social and psychological level (Berry, 2008). Another key concept here is the process of socialisation in which groups of individuals learn and adopt the behaviours of the host country (Matsumoto & Juang, 2013). Liou *et al* (2013: 615) state that acculturation is a 'complex process of adapting to a new cultural milieu and finding ways to perform in this new environment'. Behaviours are culturally defined and often considered in relation to an adaptation strategy which refers to both the process and outcome of acculturation. Evidence of how migrants acculturate to their new host country is often considered in relation to health-related outcomes, whilst the process of acculturating to the practice environment undertaken by healthcare professionals is rarely explored.

The available literature in relation to the experiences of nurses indicates that differences and variations in the performance of clinical skills and decision making are evident and cause stress and frustration (Yi & Jezewski, 2000; Omeri & Atkins, 2002; Ea *et al*, 2008). Midwives have been reported to feel a great deal of frustration and loss of professional autonomy as a result of different models of care (Davies *et al*, 2010). For midwives who migrated to Australia, for example, Sidebotham and Ahern (2011) describe the concept of *capitulation* where midwives accepted their place within the new system and relinquished their prior role. Others were reluctant to do this and detached from the models of care, leaving midwifery to find positions within public or private sectors where they felt they could fulfil their role as a midwife. In contrast, some of the midwives interviewed described ways in which they had found a comfortable space to practise as a midwife, by identifying midwives (often internationally educated) with shared philosophies. These midwives remained positive regardless of the frustrations experienced in relation to the midwifery model of care and relationships with obstetricians. These insights illustrate similar challenges to those experienced by midwives within the UK. In the absence of additional challenges presented by language issues, Sidebotham and Ahern (2011: 321) conclude: 'the assumption that midwives share identical values and beliefs about what midwifery is and the role of the midwife, and can move seamlessly between professional cultures are not supported.' Whilst the desire for a better lifestyle is a key reason for migration, the difficulties experienced in relation to acculturating into the professional environment is not diminished between countries where English is the dominant language.

Further questions regarding the experiences of midwives whose first language is not English may reveal additional challenges, especially in relation to language issues, communication styles and cultural practices. Whilst inclusivity as an overarching societal principle may support the maintenance of a strong cultural identity for migrants within the health service, the provision of support for the individual midwife to assimilate into their new cultural surroundings seems rather more challenging, especially for those who have assumed a more autonomous role elsewhere.

Interviews with midwives undertaken as part of a larger study into the equal opportunities for overseas-trained nurses and other healthcare professionals (Smith *et al,* 2006) provide insights into the negative experiences of African midwives who find difficulty in gaining promotion in their host countries. Similar findings are reported by Henry (2007) who concludes that cultural differences become institutionalised resulting in a feeling of demoralisation.

Applying a salutogenic approach

Stress as a global issue affects healthcare professionals in different ways. For migrant healthcare professionals, stress acts as a major 'push' factor for midwives to leave their home countries. Furthermore, the migration experience is also associated with the stress of working in a new country. Differences in the models of care and cultural practices are also described as factors which increase stress and dissatisfaction for migrant midwives who attempt to adapt to their host countries. It is suggested here that the application of a salutogenic model may be useful to examine how migrant midwives can cope with the stress of working within new maternity care environments with the view of promoting their health and wellbeing. Salutogenesis as a theoretical model aims to find and examine factors which act to promote and maintain health (Antonovsky, 1996).

Promoting a strong sense of coherence (SOC) (Antonovsky, 1985) is associated with reduced stress, burnout and depression. This is understood as characteristics which maintain an individual's regulation and reaction capacity for health. It is related to the individual's perception of the world around them and the resources they may call upon to cope with different stressors (Antonovsky, 1996). Generalised resistance resources (GRRs) are described as characteristics which facilitate the management of tension generated by stressors. GRRs influence the individual's perception of stressors, which also guide their SOC. On this basis we suggest that a salutogenic model could be useful to address how midwives can perceive challenging and potentially stressful situations as meaningful, manageable and comprehensible, drawing on their own resources to reduce the development of stress. During the process of acculturation, where midwives are adjusting to their new surroundings, creating a more positive approach to the working environment may be beneficial to maintain a strong sense of self, self-efficacy and cultural identity.

Multicultural practice environments

Our current knowledge suggests that midwives seek opportunities to practise midwifery across the world, thus creating a multicultural practice environment, where professionals from a number of different cultures work together. However, the available evidence, whilst limited, indicates that, for some midwives, this experience may present challenges, especially in adjusting to their new environment, particularly in relation to different models of midwifery care. It is suggested that tensions may develop between members of the workforce where cultural differences exist; these cultural differences may also appear between the workforce and the public. This may be particularly relevant to larger city-based maternity services where a more diverse multicultural workforce exists. These environments may present complex challenges for both midwives and women; many of which have not been explored in the literature. One example of a multicultural practice environment is discussed by Almutairi *et al* (2015). This research is based in Saudi Arabia where the healthcare system is dependent on health professionals from across the world. The complexity of a multicultural nursing workforce is captured by Almutairi *et al* (2015: 16) in their discussion of the position of migrant nurses:

> *Expatriate nurses working in Saudi Arabia bring different cultural values, beliefs, customs, behaviors and attitudes with them that can greatly differ from those of their patients, their Saudi Arabian employers and colleagues, and their non-Saudi colleagues. Many are employed… without the Arabic language skills that might facilitate nurse-patient and nurse-employer interactions.*

Issues of language capability and interpretation of meaning are clearly implicated as potential factors which may adversely affect the abilities of professionals to practise in a competent and safe way. The multicultural nature of the workforce may cause some conflict with the culture of the people they care for. This can result in preconceptions, discrimination and intolerance. Almutairi *et al* note that 'participants exhibited their unconscious prejudice toward the practices of Saudi people, using their own cultural background as the yardstick for all behaviour' (Almutairi *et al*, 2015: 18).

Whilst mobility presents midwives with an ideal opportunity to work in different cultural contexts, this may also reveal varying perceptions of the role of the midwife. Edwards and Glover (2010: 250), in a discussion of midwifery practice in Dubai, suggest that 'many midwives find that they are not able to practise fully within their scope and often find cultural adjustment difficult; as a result many return home after only two or three months'. A survey of pregnant women in Abu Dhabi (Edwards *et al*, 2014), revealed that there was a general lack of knowledge of the role and scope of practice of the midwife. Establishing the role of the midwife through a post-registration midwifery programme and licensing and regulation systems has contributed to the development of midwifery in Dubai, thus producing 'locally grown midwives' (Edwards & Glover, 2010: 252).

In recognition of the global role of the midwife and as a means to 'strengthen midwifery worldwide' the International Confederation of Midwives (ICM) has developed global standards for midwifery education and regulation, and essential competencies for midwifery practice (ICM, 2013):

> *Together, the ICM essential competencies and the global standards for regulation and education provide a professional framework that can be used by midwifery associations, midwifery regulators, midwifery educators and governments to strengthen the midwifery profession and raise the standard of midwifery practice in their jurisdiction. When midwives work within such a professional framework they are supported and enabled to fulfil their role and contribute fully to the delivery of maternal and newborn care in their country.* (ICM, 2011: 1)

Global standards for the initial education of professional nurses and midwives (WHO, 2009) provide a foundation for midwifery education as a means by which the variation in education across countries and continents can be reduced. Raising the standard of midwifery education provides an opportunity for countries to invest in the midwifery profession, advancing its ability to provide care for the local population of mothers and babies. It is stated that the standards 'serve as a benchmark for moving education and learning systems forward to produce a common competency-based outcome in an age of increasing globalization' (WHO, 2009: 12). Fleming *et al* (2011) developed, piloted and validated 27 scenarios based on the ICM competency statements with a group of 68 midwives from Slovenia; 58 midwives from Germany; 63 midwives from Scotland and 76 midwives from Kosovo. This research concluded that testing the scenarios with midwives across four countries demonstrated the transferrability of midwifery practice across countries, where diverse midwifery practice was known to take place. The results of this study not only support the development of global competencies for midwifery education, but also emphasise the educational value in the discussion of scenarios which reveal issues of competence across countries where the scope of practice is diverse.

The ICM's goal is to increase the global capacity of the midwifery workforce and to improve the competence of midwives. The lack of recognition and the resulting low salaries have previously been considered in this chapter as major reasons for migration from sub-Saharan countries where the skills of midwives are desperately needed. Whilst setting global standards may be seen as a way to support the migration of midwives, it has a major role in raising the status and profile of midwives within and across countries, including those within sub-Saharan Africa, thus strengthening the role and contribution of midwives.

Conclusion

Set against the background of the global mobility of healthcare professionals, this chapter has discussed some of the key issues in relation to the migration of midwives. The mobility of health professionals is driven by unsatisfactory working conditions and the lack of resources resulting in dissatisfaction and discontent. Global data suggest that this occurs in sub-Saharan countries where the mortality rates are the highest. Whilst the ICM, through the setting of global standards, is addressing the need to strengthen the role of the midwife, more needs to be done to develop maternity services within these countries to maintain their workforce and improve care. The establishment of midwifery programmes of education is seen as a way of securing a local workforce, lessening the need for individuals to migrate. In some countries it may address some of the difficulties created by the recruitment of a multicultural workforce. The ability to migrate is also a freedom which can be translated into the application of knowledge and skills between countries, thus contributing to the quality of care. The issues of risk and competence are important within the safety of healthcare, and this has been noted, especially where there are linguistic differences resulting in communication difficulties. Systems of registration and competency assessment therefore need to be transparent and will not only serve to illustrate the patterns of mobility, but also the process of seeking registration. Equally, monitoring competence and securing systems of fitness to practise are areas for further development across countries. The formation of the Network of European Midwifery Regulators (NEMIR) is a positive approach to the development of a more coherent system. However, this chapter has highlighted the ways in which midwives attempt to deal with the stress created by attempting to adapt to different work environments and models of care. The application of a salutogenic model may be useful to examine the complexity of the maternity care environment in which a focus is placed on the promotion of health and wellbeing practice. What is clearly demonstrated is the dearth of data in relation to the mobility and migration experiences of midwives. Increasing our knowledge and understanding of the process, experience and impact of the mobility of midwives will raise an awareness of the diversity of the role across countries, and the personal and professional meaning of midwifery within a cultural context while at the same time helping to promote the global significance of the midwife in the care of women and their families.

Research recommendations

Much of our current understanding of mobility and migration of midwives is derived from research with nurses and health professionals, resulting in our limited knowledge of the relationship between migration and midwifery. Furthermore, cultural differences in relation to pregnancy and childbirth necessitate the need to support international midwives. Some areas may be more challenging to explore due to the inadequate systems of registration and data collection in some countries, although it is noted that registration of nurses and midwives is well established in African countries with South Africa being the first country to establish a system of registration. However, the deficit in data presents a challenge for researchers to begin to develop a programme of research to address the following principal areas:

- The experience of midwives in relation to the registration process and competence assessment across Europe.
- An exploration of the lived experience of migrant midwives in relation to professional and personal aspects of acculturation.
- An exploration of the mobility patterns of midwives between developing countries, from developing countries to developed

countries, and between developed countries.

- The degree to which women, midwives and employers value the contribution of midwives from different cultural backgrounds.
- The degree to which a multicultural workforce influences the quality and delivery of midwifery care.
- The use of a salutogenic model to explore the experience of stress within the host maternity care environment and in strengthening migrant midwives' capacity when they return to their home countries.

From a broader European perspective:

- A European study of best practices in relation to the registration and regulation of midwives.
- An evaluation of the impact of the Network of European Midwifery Regulators on the regulation of the midwifery profession across European countries.

References

Almutairi AF, McCarthy A & Gardner G (2015). Understanding cultural competence in a multicultural nursing workforce: registered nurses' experience in Saudi Arabia. *J Transcult Nurs* 26(1): 16-23.

Antonovsky A (1985). The life cycle, mental health and the sense of coherence. *Israel J Psychiatry Relat Sci* 22: 273-280.

Antonovsky A (1996). The salutogenic model as a theory to guide health promotion. *Health Promot Int* 11(1): 11-18.

Berry JW (2008). Globalisation and acculturation. *Int J Intercult Relat 32*: 328-336.

Bourgeault IL, Neiterman E & Le Brun J (2011). Midwives on the move: comparing the requirements for practice and integration context for internationally educated midwives in Canada with the U.S., U.K. and Australia. *Midwifery* 27(3): 368-375.

Church S & Grey K (2011). Culture shift. *RCM Midwives* 6: 40-41.

Clark PF, Stewart JB & Clark DA (2006). The globalization of the labour market for health-care professionals. *Int Labour Rev* 145: 37-64.

Davies L, Kensington M, Daellenbach R & Pairman S (2010). Following the dream: the experiences of British midwives working in New Zealand. *MIDIRS Midwifery Digest* 20(2): 168-173.

Department of Health (2015). Language controls for nurses, midwives, dentists, dental care professionals, pharmacists and pharmacy technicians – proposed changes to the Dentists Act 1984, the Nursing and Midwifery Order 2001, the Pharmacy Order 2010 and the Pharmacy (Northern Ireland) Order 1976. A joint four-country wide paper for consultation. London: Department of Health.

Dunkley L & Haider S (2011). *Workforce Risks and Opportunities: Nursing and Midwifery.* London: Centre for Workforce Intelligence.

Edwards G, Crowley T, Elsori D & Sarr M (2014). What is a midwife? A survey of pregnant women in Abu Dhabi. *Pract Midwife* 17(6): 31-34.

Edwards G & Glover E (2010). Midwifery practice in Dubai. *MIDIRS Midwifery Digest* 20(2): 249-252.

Ea EE, Griffin MQ, L'Eplattenier N & Fitzpatrick JJ (2008). Job satisfaction and acculturation among Filipino registered nurses. *J Nurs Scholarsh* 40(1): 46-51.

Fleming V, Pehlke-Milde J, Davies S & Zaksek T (2011). Developing and validating scenarios to compare midwives' knowledge and skills with the International Confederation of Midwives' essential competencies in four European countries. *Midwifery* 27: 854-860.

Henry L (2007). Institutionalised disadvantage: older Ghanaian nurses' and midwives' reflections on career progression. *J Clin Nurs* 16 (12): 2196-2203.

International Confederation of Midwives (ICM) (2010). *Essential Competencies for Basic Midwifery Practice.* Revised 2013. The Hague: The Netherlands.

International Confederation of Midwives (ICM) (2011). *Global Standards for Midwifery Regulation.* The Hague: The Netherlands.

International Confederation of Midwives (ICM) (2013). *Global Standards for Midwifery Education.* The Hague: The Netherlands.

Liou S-R, Tsai H-M & Cheng CY (2013). Acculturation, collectivist orientation and organisational commitment among Asian nurses working in the US healthcare system. *J Nurs Manag* 21: 614-623.

Matsumoto D & Juang L (2013). *Culture & Psychology.* International edn. Wadsworth Publishing Co Inc.

Mills EJ, Kanters S, Hagopian A, Bansback N, Nachega J, Alberton M, Au-Yeung CG, Mtambo A, Boureault IL, Luboga S, Hogg RS & Ford N (2011). The financial cost of doctors emigrating from sub-Saharan Africa: human capital analysis. *BMJ* 343: d7031.

Network of European Midwife Regulators (NEMIR) (2009). *Survey of European Midwifery Regulators.* London: Nursing and Midwifery Council.

Network of European Midwife Regulators (NEMIR) (2010). *Survey of European Midwifery Regulators.* London: Nursing and Midwifery Council.

Nursing and Midwifery Council (NMC) (2011). *Registering as a nurse or midwife in the UK – for applicants trained within the European Union (EU) and European Economic Area (EEA).* London: Nursing and Midwifery Council.

Nursing and Midwifery Council (NMC) (2014). *Registering as a nurse or midwife in the UK – for applicants trained outside the European Union (EU) and European Economic Area (EEA).* London: Nursing and Midwifery Council.

Offermanns G, Malle EM & Jusic A (2011). Mobility, language and neighbours: Austria as source and destination country. In: Wismar M, Maier CB, Glinos IA, Dussault G & Figueras J (eds). *Health Professional Mobility and Health Systems: Evidence from 17 European countries* (Observatory Studies). First edition. England: WHO Regional Office for Europe. Chapter 4, pp89-127.

Omeri A & Atkins K (2002). Lived experiences of immigrant nurses in New South Wales, Australia: searching for meaning. *Int J Nurs Stud* 39: 495-505.

Palm W, Wismar M, Van Ginneken E, Busse R, Ernst K & Figueras J (2011). Towards a renewed Community framework for safe, high-quality and efficient cross-border health care within the European Union. In: Wismar M, Maier CB, Glinos IA, Dussault G & Figueras J (eds). *Health Professional Mobility and Health Systems: Evidence from 17 European countries* (Observatory Studies). First edition. England: WHO Regional Office for Europe. Chapter 2, pp23-46.

Sidebotham M & Ahern K (2011). Finding a way: The experiences of UK educated midwives finding their place in the midwifery workforce in Australia. *Midwifery* 27(3): 316-323.

Smith P, Allan H, Henry LW, Larsen JA, Mackintosh M (2006). *Valuing and Recognising the Talents of a Diverse Health Care Workforce.* Report of the REOH project. University of Surrey and the Open University.

Tjadens F, Wieland C & Eckert J (2012). *Mobility of Health Professionals: Health Systems, Work Conditions, Patterns of Health Workers' Mobility and Implications for Policy Makers.* Berlin and Heidelberg: Springer-Verlag.

Wismar M, Maier CB, Glinos IA, Dussault G & Figueras J (2011). *Health Professional Mobility and Health Systems Evidence from 17 European countries (Observatory Studies).* First edition. England: WHO Regional Office for Europe.

World Health Organization (WHO) (2006). *The World Health Report 2006 – Working Together for Health.* Geneva: World Health Organization.

World Health Organization (WHO) (2009). *Global Standards for the Initial Education of Professional Nurses and Midwives.* Geneva: World Health Organization.

World Health Organization (WHO) (2010). *Global Code of Practice on the International Recruitment of Health Personnel.* Sixty-third World Health Assembly-WHA63.16. Geneva: World Health Organization.

Yi M & Jezewski MA (2000). Korean nurses' adjustment to hospitals in the United States of America. *J Adv Nurs* 32, 721-729.

CHAPTER 8

Leadership development of nurses and midwives to improve maternal-child healthcare in Africa

Christa van der Walt and Karin Minnie

Introduction

This chapter provides a brief overview of the work of the Africa Maternal-Child Health Nurse Leadership Academy (MCHNLA). It also highlights the challenges midwives, in particular, face and the subsequent need for the development of leadership skills of maternal-child health nurses and midwives. Against this background the development and implementation of the Maternal-Child Health Nurse (and Midwife) Leadership Academy will be discussed from a theoretical framework based on the work of Kouzes and Posner (2013). The assessment of the South African Leadership Academy pilot will then be presented followed by an adapted model that is currently being used for the first Africa cohort of fellows from South Africa, Uganda, Malawi and Swaziland.

With this real-time experiment we wish to demonstrate how leadership development can be used as a vehicle for the transformation of maternal-child health and maternity service provision.

The need for strong leaders in maternal-child health and maternity care provision

Sub-Saharan Africa has the highest maternal and child-under-five mortality rates in the world. This region has not met Millennium Development Goals 4 and 5 in spite of the fact that some countries showed a decrease in maternal and child mortality (United Nations, 2014). The death of a mother is one of the greatest tragedies for a community and her surviving children. Child health is directly dependent on the health of the mother. Neonatal deaths constitute almost 40% of the estimated 9.7 million children-under-five deaths in the world each year and 60% of infant deaths. With more than 500,000 women dying each year in childbirth or from complications during pregnancy, babies of such mothers have a poor chance of survival compared to those babies whose mothers survive.

Although the African Union dedicated the decade 2010-2020 to women, and improving their political, social and economic standing, much still needs to be done in the field of maternal-child health – a sector where midwives and nurse-midwives play a crucial role. Nurses and midwives, because of their pivotal role in the healthcare system (Bogren et al, 2013), are in the unique position to lead healthcare transformation. Furthermore, individuals can make a difference – leadership is not just a job title, or reserved for people with authority and power, but something which can be learned (Kouzes & Posner, 2013).

Today's complex healthcare systems require good leaders at all levels (Porter-O'Grady, 2011). Porter-O'Grady (2011: 33) argues that, in general, leadership at all levels of the healthcare system is needed. To transform healthcare, and maternity care in Africa in particular, and to lead change, nurses and midwives are also required to be leaders in their daily work (Bell & Toolan, 2012: 36-37). Porter-O'Grady (2011: 33) defines a clinical leader as a health professional who is *'…a competent professional involved in providing direct and indirect clinical care, who enables oneself and influences others to improve care'*. If one adds that leadership is defined as *'creating a way for people to contribute to making something extra-ordinary happen'* (Kouzes & Posner, 2007: 3), we believe the work of the MCHNLA is crucial.

Unfortunately, many leaders are ageing and retiring soon (Sherman et al, 2013: 899; Stichler, 2013: 956). Thus, if Africa needs a transformation of maternal-child healthcare, MCH nurse and midwife leaders are needed to lead this process. Young leaders should be identified and trained as a matter of urgency to be positioned within the health sector to facilitate changes in practice. We believe that positioning MCH nurses and midwives in strong leadership positions and helping them to find their voices is one of the solutions to overcome the unacceptably high maternal, neonatal and children-under-five mortality and morbidity rates in Africa.

Maternal-Child Health Nurse Leadership Academy

Johnson & Johnson and Sigma Theta Tau International, the Honor Society of Nursing (STTI), worked in partnership with a team of specialist midwives and neonatal and child health nurses to develop the Africa Maternal-Child Health Nurse Leadership Academy (MCHNLA). The authors of this chapter were involved in the African MCHNLA from the start and are still involved as faculty lead (project manager) (CvdW) and faculty consultant (CM).

The MCHNLA is an 18-month, mentored leadership development experience. The functional unit of the Academy consists of a faculty consultant, mentor and mentee. All processes and outcomes are monitored and assessed through standardised instruments such as the Leadership Practices Inventory developed by Kouzes and Posner and narratives from faculty and dyads (STTI, 2013). A dyad refers to the mentor-mentee pair.

The MCHNLA develops the leadership competencies of nurses and midwives who have worked in a variety of healthcare settings in the USA over the past two decades, and now in South Africa, Malawi, Uganda and Swaziland. The Africa MCHNLA was successfully piloted in the North-West Province of South Africa during 2012-2013. The Academy prepares maternal-child health nurses and midwives to effectively lead inter-professional teams to improve the quality of healthcare for childbearing women, and children up to five years of age. The MCHNLA in general and the Africa MCHNLA believe that enhancing the leadership capabilities of MCH nurses and midwives has the potential to transform maternal-child healthcare in Africa.

Theoretical framework

The leadership skills component of the Academy is based on the research of Jim Kouzes and Barry Posner which is described in their book *The Leadership Challenge®* (Kouzes & Posner, 2013). The Kouzes and Posner (KP) model proposes that leadership is a measurable, learnable, and teachable set of behaviours (Kouzes & Posner, 2013) (see Table 1). The Academy believes that nurses and midwives can learn these behaviours most effectively by applying them in a clinical setting. The programme was developed to put these learned behaviours into action by assisting and supporting the mentee in developing and implementing an evidence-based project that is centred on improving the quality of maternal-child health outcomes and maternal-child nursing and midwifery practice.

Table 1:

The principles of the KP model (Kouzes & Posner, 2013)

1. Model the way by clarifying values and finding one's voice whilst affirming shared values by setting the example;
2. Inspire a shared vision – this entails envisioning the future by imagining exciting and ennobling possibilities, and enlisting others in a common vision by appealing to shared aspirations;
3. Challenge the process, which refers to the search for opportunities by seizing the initiative and by looking outwards for innovative ways to improve, and experimenting and taking risks by constantly generating small wins and learning from experience;
4. Enable others to act by fostering collaboration through building trust and facilitating relationships, and strengthening others by increasing self-determination and developing competence; and
5. Encourage the heart – this principle refers to recognising contributions by showing appreciation for individual excellence, and celebrating the values and victories by creating a spirit of community.

Leadership competencies of maternal-child health nurses and midwives are developed through:

1. A workshop series facilitated by the faculty consultants
2. Mentor-mentee pairs where one-on-one mentoring by more experienced mentors takes place
3. A leadership challenge / quality improvement project
4. Presentation of posters of mentees' projects at the annual conference of the Tau Lambda Chapter-at-Large or the Biennial Convention of

Sigma Theta Tau International Honor Society of Nursing (STTI)

5. Ongoing access to an STTI online MCH community (STTI, 2014).

Educational approach towards leadership development

The functional unit of the Academy consists of a triad, consisting of a mentee, mentor and faculty consultant. The mentee and mentor are paired with an expert faculty consultant, preferably a doctoral-qualified faculty, who acts as a facilitator during the mentee's leadership journey. This triad works collaboratively towards attaining the mentee's leadership development goals.

Recruitment of dyads

The process of recruitment in the North American cohorts is based on the mentee identifying an expert mentor who participates in the Academy workshops and guides the mentee through the leadership development journey. This process was adapted for the Africa MCHNLA by using a top-down recruitment strategy. Together with stakeholders, faculty advisers identified persons in current leadership positions who could mentor maternal-child health nurses and midwives. The faculty consultants and the mentors identify young and upcoming leaders in their regions. The reason for this approach is based on the African principles of respect for leaders and the still inherent hierarchies in nursing and midwifery.

The mentor is an individual who is not the mentee's direct supervisor, but who is familiar with the mentee's practice setting, agrees to champion, advise, and advocate for the mentee, and demonstrates the leadership characteristics required of a mentor. The mentor supports the mentee through his or her leadership journey whilst the mentee develops a quality improvement (QI) project that is focused on improving maternal-child health outcomes and maternal-child nursing or midwifery practice. These QI projects must address an area of concern to the particular setting or community and must be evidence-based, for example, the implementation of kangaroo mother care or of neuro-developmental care practices. As part of the project development, the mentee forms an inter-professional team in his or her practice setting or community to develop his/her project.

A faculty consultant is a doctoral-qualified midwife, neonatal nurse or child health nurse specialist. The faculty consultants are each assigned to one or two mentee/mentor pair(s) (dyads) and assist with personal leadership development, team development, and project planning, implementation and evaluation. A team of faculty consultants develop the Academy curriculum and present the workshops.

The Africa MCHNLA

In 2009, the STTI Honor Society for Nurses approached nurse and midwifery leaders from a variety of African countries to discuss the possible roll-out to Africa. From many experiences in the past, it is known that only a few of these initiatives have been adapted successfully in Africa. After a call for proposals, the North-West University (NWU) in South Africa was granted funding to pilot the MCHNLA in the North-West Province of South Africa (STTI, 2013).

The Africa version of the STTI Maternal-Child Health Nurse Leadership Academy is built on this pilot that was run for 18 months in South Africa. Six dyads took part in this pilot. Five faculty consultants from the School of Nursing Science of the NWU were chosen as leadership candidates. With the help of a team of stakeholders, we selected four mentors from the public health sector and one from the private sector. The mentors were then advised on choosing their mentees.

With the help of an experienced leadership counsellor, the team of faculty consultants worked together to adapt the North American curriculum to fit the needs of maternal-child health and maternity care in South Africa. Not only did we need to adapt the language to South African English as none of the faculty or the dyad pairs were English speaking, but we also adapted the process, case studies and metaphors used during the workshops. The mentees, together with their mentors and faculty consultants, selected projects to address issues of concern at their workplaces. The mentees were also assisted to promote their projects to the leadership of their organisations, one of the skills they had to master.

Quality improvement projects on kangaroo mother care, discharge planning for parents of preterm infants, community-based interventions to improve early antenatal care and follow-up of children of HIV-positive mothers, the use of the partogram and the prevention of postpartum haemorrhage were implemented successfully. All of these initiatives are still running and three of them have now been adopted by the provincial Department of Health. All mentees have been promoted and one is working towards a Master's degree in Midwifery and Neonatal Nursing. Fellows from the pilot Academy started a Facebook group, Midwives on Fire, and are instrumental in the transformation of maternity care at their workplaces. The kangaroo care unit that was established is still going strong and has even expanded, while a midwifery symposium, which was an activity developed as part of continuous education by one of the dyads, expanded to become an annual provincial symposium for midwives and neonatal nurses, supported by the provincial Department of Health.

The South African pilot showed that the MCHNLA can be successfully adopted and implemented in Africa and, although the Africa Academy is a work in progress, the preliminary results show a clear impact on both mentors' and mentees' leadership competencies, and on the quality of care in settings where mentees implemented their leadership challenge projects. The immediate effect of interventions in the dyads' work place strengthened the relationships between the Academy, the NWU, the Department of Health and the community.

After the South African pilot finished, the first Africa cohort of 12 dyads started their 18-month leadership journey in 2014 with funding and support from Johnson & Johnson and STTI. Five dyads and three faculty consultants from Malawi, Uganda and Swaziland, and a further six faculty consultants and seven dyads from the Limpopo, Free State, North West and Gauteng provinces in South Africa were included in this first cohort. The majority of the dyads operate in public hospitals and clinics and one dyad works in a private hospital.

The 2014-2015 cohort implemented their QI projects on helping babies breathe, improving the administration of magnesium sulphate to prevent eclamptic convulsions, the implementation of neuro-developmental best practice guidelines in a specialist neonatal intensive care unit, the promotion of appropriate use of the partogram in a private hospital, and improving intrapartum fetal observation.

Programme evaluation

An external company extensively evaluates the programme. The objectives of the evaluation are to (a) document the evidence of changes in mentees' and mentors' leadership-related knowledge, skills, and behaviours, as well as evidence of organisational and/or patient impact from mentee projects; (b) summarise mentees' and mentors' feedback on the workshops and on the MCHNLA as a whole; and (c) identify aspects of the evaluation instruments and data collection processes that could be improved for the next cohort.

Various standardised instruments (see Table 2) are administered during the course of the Academy and follow-up measurements are taken. These instruments measure the mentees' and mentors' leadership practices, knowledge and skills, behaviour and satisfaction with the workshops. At the conference the mentees' posters are evaluated, as well as the impact their projects have had on health professionals, mothers and babies and the communities (STTI, 2013).

Table 2:

Evaluation areas of measure

PARTICIPANT IMPACT	ORGANISATIONAL IMPACT	HEALTH NETWORK IMPACT	PATIENT IMPACT
• Knowledge • Skills (leadership, other) • On-the-job behaviour (application of skills) • Career changes • Involvement in broader field	• Efficiency of individual agency processes • Broader systems efficiency • Cost efficiency/ change to cost of services • Clinical practice (clinical policies and behaviours) • Service availability • Number of patients/ clients served • Service quality • Financial health of organisation	• Availability of care/treatment in community • Overall number/per cent of community members served • Quality of care/ treatment • Cost of care/ treatment • Network-wide process efficiency • Patient uptake of services (% of service needs met in particular health issue areas) • Patient satisfaction • Patient behavioural or biological indicators • Prevalence of targeted health conditions (morbidity, mortality)	• Patient uptake of services (% of service needs met in particular health issue areas) • Patient satisfaction • Patient behavioural or biological indicators • Prevalence of targeted health conditions (morbidity, mortality)

During the pilot Academy a steady increase in leadership knowledge, skills and behaviour was found in both the mentee and mentor groups. Although the pilot was a steep learning curve for the faculty, never before having participated in such an intervention, the dyads were satisfied with the workshops and in particular voiced their appreciation for the opportunity to participate in the Academy (STTI, 2013). The same trend is seen in the current cohort's measurements. Faculty consultants are more confident about changing the North American curriculum, resulting in a shared feeling of ownership. Continuous feedback from participants and one another at the end of each day of the two workshops in 2014 and 2015 helps us to immediately respond to special requests such as using case scenarios constructed by the dyads rather than the ones in the planned programme. We also used more role-play and interactive sessions where mentees took the lead in facilitating sessions (STTI, 2013, 2015). The full evaluation of the first cohort of the 2014-2015 Africa MCHNLA is currently under way.

To date, there have been 86 mentor/mentee pairs in the United States and Canada and 18 from Africa. The faculty have created and implemented healthcare projects and programmes to positively affect maternal-child practice and outcomes (STTI, 2014).

Conclusion

The MCHNLA could successfully be adapted from the North American model, and early findings of the battery of instruments used to measure the process and outcomes of the Academy showed that leadership development of maternal-child health nurses and midwives can improve the health of mothers, babies and children under five. There is a substantial impact on the skills, knowledge and practice of the dyads as well as on the health of mothers, babies and the communities. For example, where communities were targeted, awareness-raising led to an increase in early antenatal attendance (MCHNLA, 2014/2015).

The success of a venture such as the Africa MCHNLA requires the continuous commitment of funders. Johnson & Johnson and the STTI Honor Society of Nursing made the Africa MCHNLA possible. The Leadership Academy is expensive and in future additional funding will be required. With more funding and resources more communities can be reached and more mothers and babies can be saved.

We, Christa van der Walt and Karin Minnie, were part of the initial planning in 2009, participated as faculty consultants in the South African Pilot and are still involved as faculty lead (CvdW) and faculty consultant (KM) in the current Africa MCHNLA. As faculty consultants and faculty lead our own leadership competency developed as we started using these principles in our daily work life. Being part of the Leadership Academy gives us the opportunity to see how the mentors and mentees find their voices, and gain confidence in public speaking and project management skills. We will also act as coaches for a further roll-out of the Academy in Africa.

References

Bell M & Toolan B (2012). Leadership. *WIN* 19(10): 36-37.

Bogren MU, Van Teijlingen E & Berg M (2013). Where midwives are not yet recognized: a feasibility study of professional midwives in Nepal. *Midwifery* 29(10): 1103-1109.

Kouzes JM & Posner BZ (2013). The leadership challenge. 5th edn. San Francisco: Jossey-Boss publishers.

Maternal-Child Health Nurse Leadership Academy (McHNLA) 2014/2015: www.sttiafrica.com/mchnla/cohort-2.

Porter-O'Grady T (2011). Leadership at all levels. *Nurs Manag* 42(5): 32-37.

Sherman RC, Chiang-Hanisko L, Koszalinski R (2013). The ageing nursing workforce: a global challenge. *J Nurs Manag* 21(7): 899-902.

Sigma Theta Tau International Honor Society of Nursing (STTI) (2013). South African pilot of MCHNLA: Final Evaluation Report. Unpublished. Indianapolis: STTI.

Sigma Theta Tau International Honor Society for Nursing (STTI) (2014). The Maternal-Child Health Nurse Leadership Academy: Executive summary. Indianapolis: STTI.

Stichler JF (2013). Healthy work environments for the ageing nursing workforce. *J Nurs Manag* 21: 956-963.

United Nations (2014). The Millennium Development Goals Report 2014. Available from: www.un.org/millenniumgoals/2014%20MDG%20report/MDG%202014%20English%20web.pdf

CHAPTER 9

Reflections on 'Getting Europe into Switzerland and Switzerland into Europe'

Swiss participation in COST Action ISCH 0907 from 2010 to 2014

Ans Luyben, Claudia Meier Magistretti, Barbara Kaiser, Iréne Maffi and Annette Kuhn

Introduction

Optimal maternal and infant health is critical to effective parenting, societal wellbeing, resource use, and economic growth. Therefore all countries in Europe aim to maximise the safety and wellbeing of about 4.7 million women in childbirth each year (Downe, 2009). However, significant cross-national differences in maternity care cultures, philosophies, organisation, provision and outcomes have been noticed, which are affecting the United Nations' Millennium Development Goals 4 and 5. On the one hand, underprovision of care for marginalised groups, such as migrants, still continues, whereas on the other hand, overprovision of medical care in privileged populations takes place. European rates of caesarean sections are over 80% in some hospitals, with Italy having the highest overall rate in the world, at 38% (Downe, 2009). In 2009, a group of European researchers agreed that these differences called for an interdisciplinary, collaborative research approach in order to scope the nature of maternity care provision, and to determine the effects on women and families in order to develop innovative methods for disseminating insights from excellent systems of provision (Downe, 2009).

As a result of their initiative, COST Action IS 0907 'Childbirth Cultures, Concerns and Consequences' was proposed and accepted by COST Europe in December 2009 (Downe, 2009). The Action aimed to advance scientific knowledge about ways of improving maternity care provision and outcomes for mothers, babies and families across Europe by understanding what works, for whom, and in what circumstances, and by identifying and learning from the best. During its course, more than 23 European countries, as well as China, Australia and South Africa, were involved. In order to achieve the aims of the Action, the work took place in five working groups, which were:

1. Organisational systems design and culture
2. Outcome measurement (clinical, psychological and socio-cultural)
3. Impact on migrant women
4. Techniques for identifying the best in complex systems
5. Innovative knowledge transfer and translation.
6. As a result of the multidisciplinary collaboration a variety of approaches, in particular complexity theory and salutogenesis, were used.

The Action ran over a period of four years, from 2010 to 2014. Ever since its start, a multidisciplinary Swiss team participated in the Action. This chapter addresses how the Swiss team participated in and contributed to this Action, which included three core studies that explored childbirth cultures and concerns, and looks at the consequences in Switzerland within its framework.

Background

Country profile

Situated in Central Europe, Switzerland is a federalist country, consisting of 23 cantons and 3 'half-cantons'. The population consists of approximately 8.1 million people, who speak four formal languages: German (or 'Swiss-German'), French, Italian and Rhaeto-Romanic. In 2013, 23.7%

of this population were migrants (SFSO, 2015). The federalist structure of the country means that most governing responsibility is left with the cantons, who in turn might delegate some to the municipalities. So while a central, national government is in place, multiple decisions are taken at a decentralised level. Thus Federal Law regulates little healthcare organisation and provision.

The Swiss healthcare system is second on the global list of the most expensive healthcare systems and is the most expensive in Europe (AngloInfo, 2015). Healthcare expenditure is high, taking up 10.8% of the GDP (Esmail, 2013). Health insurance has only been obligatory since 1996 and certain healthcare packages are defined within the Federal Law (De Graeve *et al*, 2001). The cantons and municipalities have a high degree of independence in the regulation and provision of care (European Observatory on Health Care Systems, 2000). Health insurance companies are important partners in the organisation of healthcare and are organised at both national and cantonal level.

Maternity care

In 2013, the birth rate in Switzerland was 10.2 per 1000 people (SFSO, 2015). The Europeristat report (Zeitlin, Mohangoo & Delnord, 2010) reported a perinatal mortality rate of 4.3 and a maternal mortality rate of 5.5 per 100,000 births. Switzerland had one of the lowest rates of mothers under 20 years of age (1.1%), but one of the highest rates of mothers of foreign origin (41.1%) in Europe. Records showed there were 3.6 physicians per 1,000 people; however these figures did not differentiate between general practitioners and specialists (Esmail, 2013; OECD, 2011). The number of nurses was reported as 14.4 and the number of midwives was estimated at 3.5 per 1,000 population (Esmail, 2013; OECD, 2011; SHV, 2014).

Whereas the state is responsible for the regulation and accreditation of medical personnel, regulation of other healthcare personnel lies with the cantons (European Observatory on Health Care Systems, 2000). While midwives are viewed as paramedical healthcare personnel in most cantons, they are regulated by cantonal law. Most midwives are employed by a hospital, while a few work independently, in a midwifery practice or in a birth centre. General practitioners have their own practices or are organised in group practices. Medical specialists are employed by a hospital, within which they might have their own practice. A larger number are, however, providing care in a private practice. For birth, clients might be referred to one of the public hospitals or a private hospital, in which the client with an independent medical doctor can use its personnel and facilities (*Belegarzt*). Healthcare providers are contracted by the insurance companies. Swiss clients of healthcare have a free choice of care provider, either a generalist or a specialist. About 90% of pregnant women attend antenatal care with their gynaecologist, who they will have visited for gynaecological care and family planning prior to their pregnancy (Luyben *et al*, 2013). During the last five years, pregnant women have become increasingly interested in care models, in which antenatal care is shared between gynaecologists and midwives, for reasons of continuity of care during childbirth and the postnatal period (Luyben *et al*, 2013). Obstetric risk selection hardly ever takes place during pregnancy, i.e., differentiation between 'low risk' (primary care; led by midwife or general practitioner) and 'high risk' (secondary care; led by gynaecologist) conditions (DeVries *et al*, 2001; Luyben & Gross, 2001). Some insurance companies offer a healthcare model with a limited choice of care providers or a 'gate keeper model', like the ones provided in the Netherlands or the United Kingdom, against reduced insurance costs care.

In 2010, at the start of the COST Action, it was noticed that the situation in maternity care, and related problems such as the high caesarean section rates, had a low priority on the Swiss agenda, both in politics and research. The reasons for this were unclear, but some assumptions could be made. On the one hand, women's issues had been of high importance in the 1990s, but seemed to have disappeared from the political agenda, possibly due to an increased need for financial savings as a result of the banking crisis of 2008. On the other hand, compared to other countries, quality of health in Switzerland was generally high, and therefore maternity care issues were not considered to be a priority.

However, since the beginning of the 2000s, the use of technology and medical interventions during childbirth has also increased in Switzerland, resulting in an increased caesarean section rate, which is up to 43% in some regions. The proportion of births without obstetrical intervention (vaginal birth without induction, forceps, ventouse or episiotomy) was only 34.8% in Switzerland in 2010: 0.7% of births took place at home, 1.5% in a birthing home and 97.8% in a hospital (SFSO, 2013). In contrast to this, possible overmedicalisation had become an issue, and the maternity care system was struggling to adequately meet the needs of the increasing migrant population. During the last decade, therefore, critical voices questioning this situation have increased.

Research in maternity care

Traditionally, research in maternity care in Switzerland has been dominated by the biomedical sciences, in particular medicine and epidemiology. On the other hand, a variety of streams, in sociology, psychology, public health and anthropology, have been addressing a diversity of aspects of becoming a mother, early child development and organisational system design and cultures from different perspectives. Little attention has been paid so far to this research as little exchange has taken place between the biomedical and humanistic disciplines. Thus the biomedical disciplines have remained the dominant discipline in maternity care research and funding acquisition. Research is traditionally funded by the Swiss National Fund (SNF) or one of the many Swiss foundations and charities. Most research takes place in university settings, which are governed and financed by state institutions.

This situation changed with a national decision in 2004 to move the (college) education of healthcare professionals into higher (university) education (Oertle Bürki, 2008), which meant they also had to do research in order to create their own body of knowledge. The development of these practice-orientated, academic disciplines, such as midwifery, within the universities of applied sciences therefore called for new perspectives on research in the healthcare field. However, the universities of applied sciences are largely financed by the individual cantons, with little state contribution. Additionally, they are also strongly influenced by disciplinary philosophies of economics and technology, with a market-driven approach. Within this approach, organisational system design and culture as well as consumers' views were considered to be important topics, but national knowledge about these topics appeared to be very limited. Creating this body of knowledge called, in particular, for a collaborative approach with different perspectives from a variety of involved disciplines. The framework of COST Action IS 0907 seemed to support this development, and this played a major role in encouraging Swiss participation in the Action.

Swiss participation in COST Action ISCH 0907

COST is an instrument for supporting scientific networking between member countries of the European Union (EU). While Switzerland is not an EU member, educational and scientific governmental bodies in Switzerland are supporting Swiss participation in European COST Actions, which is directed through the Swiss SBFI COST Office (head: Dr. Eva M. Klaper). On the one hand, this means that Switzerland contributes financially to COST Europe. On the other hand, Swiss applicants are financed for their participation in meetings by COST Europe. In addition to this, COST Switzerland provides opportunities for funding some collaborative projects as well as international meetings taking place in Switzerland. In order to participate, Swiss researchers have to submit an official application, which has to be approved by several Swiss governmental bodies. In the next sections, a few aspects of the Swiss participation will be highlighted, starting with the invitation.

Invitation

In Summer 2009, the first author, who had just finished her doctoral study in midwifery, health and social sciences in the United Kingdom (UK) (Luyben, 2008), was invited through her science network by the principal investigator (Professor Soo Downe) to participate in a proposal to be sent in for the annual Call for Actions from the European COST Office in Brussels. She had just accepted a position to build up a unit for midwifery research within the Health Department of a university of applied sciences. The aims of the Action were consistent with the research objectives of this unit and thus participation was viewed as supporting its development.

The proposal was well received by peer reviewers and, in November 2009, we were informed that it was close to being accepted. At the same time, we were invited to apply with a Statement of Interest to be sent to COST Switzerland. In order to fulfil the criteria, another management member and two substitutes from different disciplines working in this research field had to be located.

Application

The Statement of Interest required both a description of expected, future projects and a statement with regard to the meaning of this Action for Switzerland and Swiss researchers. While COST Action IS 0907 expected an interdisciplinary approach, the Swiss national context also required a multi-language representation. Representatives for research in the field of maternity care were recruited through several channels. As a result, the representation firstly involved a psychologist, who was connected with a large network of researchers in public health, sociology and psychology, secondly, a midwife with a doctorate in psychology connected to a wide network in French-speaking Switzerland and, thirdly, an experienced gynaecologist and researcher, with national and international connections to gynaecologists and obstetricians. The application was accepted in January 2010.

Co-ordination

The Swiss process of applying for and getting approval for a Statement of Interest places the main applicants, and the first and second Management Members (MC) in particular, in a unique situation. This means that they are primarily representing Switzerland in this Action, which involves all Swiss researchers, rather than their own institution. Thus, they have an overview of who is who in this field, and what research is needed, in order to bring 'Switzerland into Europe'. All new Swiss participants have to access the Action by contacting the Swiss MC members. In addition, the Swiss MC members are expected to disseminate all information from the COST Action amongst involved Swiss researchers, and thus bring 'Europe into Switzerland'. The expected activities underpin this focus on co-ordination, such as providing regular annual meetings for nationally involved researchers, and co-ordinating national information on an electronic and personal basis. A particularly important part of this process is the production of annual reports for the Swiss COST office, which describe work on individual proposals and projects, and the national and international networking of all the Swiss researchers and institutions involved, either within or beyond the framework of the COST Action. The COST office thus aims to monitor the increase in collaboration between international and national researchers studying the same topics. Whereas such co-ordination is challenging due to the competitive elements in the research field, this is even more so in a federalist structure, involving institutions with varying research status. Thus we learnt a lot about international and national organisational cultures in this Action, both in maternity care and in research in the French, Italian and German-speaking regions. The kind support offered by experts from both COST Switzerland and EU Research for all our activities has been memorable.

Collaboration: bringing Switzerland into Europe

COST is about international interdisciplinary collaboration in science and technology, which means that it is expected that working together, instead of alone, on specific subjects results in more and better outputs. The first COST IS0907 meeting took place in Preston (UK) in September 2010, during which Working Groups (WGs) were established and agreements on collaboration were made. We tried to participate in all five working groups, in order to provide information to other Swiss researchers. Additionally, one Swiss MC member was involved in the overall Action as Financial Rapporteur, and another as lead of the Early Stage Researchers' (ESR) group.

A national web-based platform was set up for all Swiss participation in the Action. Following this first meeting, an invitation was sent to various Swiss researchers, who might be interested in the Action, and in particular the new midwifery research units. The reactions were less positive than we thought. Some did not have time to join, some did not want to join as it was not paid as a project, some postponed their decision, and some were afraid to collaborate and to commit.

However, during the course of the Action, starting at the end of year two, trust in the Action grew, and initiatives for collaboration slowly increased within and between institutions, between language regions as well as between Swiss and international institutions. For example, collaboration with an economics department at a university resulted from participation in two proposals for EU calls. Some collaborative projects with other institutions were realised on a national level, in particular with the large-scale involvement of professional and consumer organisations (see the section on *Three studies*). The participation of new disciplines, such as anthropology, at the end of year three provided access to established networks with experienced researchers, who brought new perspectives. We aimed to have at least one Swiss participant in each of the working groups, but this took longer than expected. On the other hand, the multidisciplinary character of the COST Action helped us to overcome some traditional inter-professional problems, such as in obstetrics and midwifery.

Dissemination: bringing Europe into Switzerland

Lots of efforts were undertaken to disseminate and promote Swiss participation in the COST Action (Luyben, 2010; Luyben, 2011; Luyben *et al*, 2011). The fact that midwifery and other healthcare professions had just started to develop as new research disciplines supported these initiatives. Thus, the COST Action provided a vehicle to promote the 'product' on the market, to underpin requests for the funding of projects and to reach out to other disciplines for collaboration.

The COST Action was promoted at several national conferences in order to highlight the research efforts of both the Action and the individual research units; either as a poster, flyer or presentation. Several articles were written in professional journals on participation in the COST Action or a specific topic linked to the Action. As a consequence, this meant that it was possible to seek partners in affiliated disciplines and to promote the profile of research in specific organisations. Information from the COST meetings was electronically disseminated amongst participants.

The COST meeting in Switzerland in April 2012, followed by a national symposium, has been one of the highlights of Swiss participation. The meeting allowed Swiss researchers to network and participate in the working groups. The symposium provided a platform for promoting the topic of salutogenesis in early life, supported by international experts, national dissemination and beginning the establishment of Communities in Practice in this area (White *et al*, 2014).

The Short Term Scientific (STS) Missions of the COST Action have been another important vehicle for national dissemination and international collaboration. There was great interest from Swiss researchers to visit international experts in their institutions and for international researchers to visit Swiss institutions. In this way, new topics, such as bullying and organisational culture, were developed in Switzerland, while Swiss researchers brought their knowledge into other countries. Thus, multiple individual and institutional collaborations were developed. However, the unfavourable exchange rate of the Swiss franc, and thus the high costs of staying in Switzerland, were a barrier to several incoming STS Missions.

Additionally Swiss participation in international projects increased, and joint projects developed between Swiss members, as well as between Swiss researchers and international partners. Three such studies will be presented as examples in the next section.

Three studies

The assumption underpinning COST Action IS0907 was that the quality of professional care during pregnancy, childbirth and the postnatal period has short and long-term consequences on the health of mothers, babies and their families. In Switzerland, postnatal depression, and child negligence and abuse, are important health problems that are linked to care during this period. Whereas medical and epidemiological data are routinely collected in Switzerland, for example, by the Swiss Federal Statistical Office of the Department of Health, little knowledge was available either about the experiences of women and their new families or organisational system design and cultures (Frith *et al,* 2014). Therefore international comparison between COST partners was not possible. On top of this, adequate instruments to explore these experiences, and women's views, were lacking. The research of the Swiss participants to this Action between 2010 and 2014 therefore focused on building knowledge in these specific topic areas. Three of these studies are presented below.

MatHeR-ch.ch; Maternal Health Experiences Research during Childbirth in Switzerland (CH)

The first study 'MatHER-ch.ch' explored maternal health experiences during childbirth in Switzerland, both in regard to quality of professional care as well as the quality of health that women experienced (Burkhardt *et al,* 2013; Luyben *et al,* 2013; Luyben *et al,* 2014). The study was carried out by researchers at the Bern University of Applied Sciences, with Dr. Ans Luyben as the principal investigator. The study had been designed at the start of the COST Action and was funded by the research fund of Bern University of Applied Sciences. The study took place between May 2011 and May 2013 and used a mixed methods approach. This pilot study was carried out in three Swiss German-speaking cantons – Bern, Graubünden and Zug. Four practice partners were involved – three centres for mother-father counselling and one private gynaecological practice.

In a first step, the Maternal Experiences Survey (MES) questionnaire from Public Health Canada was translated and adapted (Chalmers *et al,* 2008). This questionnaire consisted of 300 questions on 26 topics, such as mode of birth, place of care, and breastfeeding. In a second step, this questionnaire was piloted in a survey and complementary one-to-one interviews by midwives took place with 61 women 8 to 12 months after giving birth to their child.

Participation in the study was high. Women were particularly interested in taking part in the interviews in order to tell their stories, reflect on their experience and ask the midwives any remaining questions they had. They generally expressed high satisfaction with the medical care provided, but were dissatisfied with the information and psychosocial care that they had received.

During childbirth, 98% of the women reported interventions. About one third of the women were induced; many were dissatisfied with this experience, and emphasised the need to change this management of their care. Women also reported on the fragmentation of care and the need to improve continuity of care. Due to the lack of continuity of care, (male) partners were the most important source of support during childbirth and the postnatal period. Related to this, about 15% of the women interviewed 8 to 12 months after birth reported both physical as well as psychosocial health complications, which implies that one in six women in Switzerland would be affected.

Quality and gaps in postnatal care

The second study on quality and needs in postnatal care was undertaken between November 2011 and November 2013 (Meier Magistretti *et al*, 2013; Meier Magistretti *et al*, 2014a). The main reason for undertaking this study was the decade long debate between maternity care professionals and politicians about the need to improve and expand postnatal care, although statistics produced thus far did not offer the necessary evidence to do so. Another reason was the introduction of the Swiss Diagnosis Related Groups (DRGs), which changed the reimbursement of maternity care costs. Following this, insurance companies reimbursed healthcare costs at a (lower) flat rate linked to a specific diagnosis ('birth'), and not based on the course of an individual case as previously. As a result, the the postnatal stay in hospital was reduced. Dr. Claudia Meier Magistretti and her team conducted the study. The study was collaboratively designed during the first year of the COST Action and was funded by Lucerne University of Applied Sciences and Arts.

The National Childbirth Trust in the UK had carried out a postnatal survey in 2010, and allowed us to use their questionnaire (Newburn & Bhavnani, 2010). This questionnaire was translated and adapted to the Swiss system, and launched as an online survey with 28 questions. Recruitment of the women took place through professional associations including midwives, mother-counsellors, obstetricians, Wir Eltern, and Present-Service (Zug). A survey of the French and Italian-speaking population was proposed but did not come to fruition.

Between November 2011 and December 2012 1055 women, who had given birth in 2011 and 2012 in the German-speaking regions of Switzerland, took part. Sixty-five per cent of the women had given birth to a first child. The majority of the women (74%) had given birth in hospital, 19% gave birth with a known midwife, 3% gave birth in a birth centre, and 4% at home.

Thirty two per cent of the women had experienced a complication during childbirth.

Swiss women were highly satisfied with the quality of postnatal care; this rate was higher than in the United Kingdom. The satisfaction of the women appeared to be related to the place of birth. Criticism related to time pressure and stress faced by personnel in the hospitals and inconsistency of information, mainly in regard to breastfeeding practices.

Eighty-five percent of women were of the opinion that continuity of care was very important, and stressed the need for continuity of care by a known midwife. The need for improvements in care was particularly highlighted by women who had experienced complications during childbirth. Only 48% mentioned that their care plan had been co-ordinated with them, which means that half of these women were not actively involved in the provision of their care. In an extension of the survey work, a secondary analysis of the data focused on the experiences of women who had experienced a stillbirth (Meier Magistretti, Rabhi-Sidler *et al*, 2014).

Giving birth at CHUV

The third study was called 'Giving birth at the CHUV in Lausanne', a hospital in the French-speaking part of Switzerland, and focused on the experiences of couples from antenatal classes on their return back home post birth. The research involved studying ideas, discourses and experiences of couples and maternity care providers. Professor Iréne Maffi and her team conducted the study, which was carried out at the time that she joined in the COST Action, during its third year (Maffi, 2013). The study was developed as a consequence of previous studies on this topic in countries in the Middle East, with Professor Maffi being referred to the Swiss COST Group via the Swiss COST office.

The study had an ethnographic approach and involved two stages. During the first stage, antenatal classes were attended in order to understand the interactions in these specific settings, to study the content of the classes and to listen to the discourse of the couples. This stage also involved interviews with the midwives responsible for the courses and attendance at several meetings of the team in charge of childbirth classes. During the second stage, interviews with couples were conducted, during pregnancy, immediately after birth and some months after their return back home with the baby. In addition, regular field work (observations and interviews) was carried out in the maternity hospital working with three teams, respectively, of the delivery unit and of the two postnatal services.

The study ran over two years. The preliminary conclusions were that couples were generally not very well informed about the possibility of giving birth in places other than the hospital. They were socialised in a risk culture generated by frequent and invasive medical surveillance during pregnancy. Most of them were not aware of their rights to choose the way in which they would give birth. As a consequence they gave birth in a highly technocratic setting, transforming the event into a medical procedure they underwent rather than actively lived. They experienced fear and anxieties during all the processes from pregnancy to postpartum. In addition, rigid protocols were applied to mothers and newborns making them passive recipients of medical acts. Thus, the whole process gave the impression that the development of parents' self-confidence, as well as their social and personal resources, was inhibited, rather than supported and strengthened.

The preliminary results were communicated to the hospital teams involved in the study and discussed with them. However, the study was intended to be an anthropological work on the socio-cultural aspects of the current birthing system in Switzerland rather than an evaluation of the services. As a result, a fruitful and hopefully long-standing collaboration with the department of gynaecology and obstetrics of the hospital has been established. Masters and PhD students are still doing fieldwork in the hospital, regularly communicating the results of their study to the staff. The aim is to offer a different perspective on their daily relational and material work, while allowing birth attendants to develop a different understanding of their interactions with the patients, and of their practices and, in so doing, to reflect on the current organisational culture.

Further results

The results of the studies, as described above, have contributed to national knowledge about maternity care and have fed back into the Action in order to facilitate an international comparison and contribute to a larger European discussion about childbirth cultures, best practices and their consequences on women, their children and their families. The use of the questionnaires that are routinely used in other countries allowed an international comparison of data. While the call for personalised medicine and individual care increases internationally, assessments of consumers' experiences are also of national importance. The studies that are described above have all resulted in follow-up studies, some as participative implementation studies in hospitals, some of which involved the participative design of maternity care models.

The Action, and its associated projects, resulted in a large number of publications and presentations, which have been created as outputs within the framework of this COST Action or 'beyond' this framework.

a. Within the framework of COST Action IS 0907 the following outputs were produced:

- Eight publications: three in peer-reviewed journals, three in professional journals and two book contributions
- Seventeen presentations, either oral or poster presentations. One of them was awarded with a first poster prize (Gillen, Brailey & Luyben, 2012) and one for best oral presentation (Meier Magistretti & Downe *et al*, 2014)

b. 'Beyond' the framework, several contributions were made by individual researchers and institutions:

- Seven publications: two in peer-reviewed journals, six in professional journals, and two published reports
- Twenty-five presentations, either oral or poster presentations. Two were awarded with a poster prize.

Discussion and conclusion

For Switzerland, this Action has provided a nurturing environment to develop a network of researchers aiming to explore childbirth cultures, concerns and consequences abroad as well as 'at home'. Concurrently, the ongoing international and interdisciplinary exchange with experts and early stage researchers on a European level facilitated a reflexive view from outside, which has been both nurturing and challenging.

Overall, the Action has shown added value for Swiss participation in terms of:

- Building a sustainable interdisciplinary network that will continue after the end of the Action into the planned European Maternity

Research Network. To date, 13 Swiss institutions have been participating in the network. During the course of the Action these institutions have established collaborations with 13 universities abroad. Some of these collaborations are ongoing, both nationally as well as internationally.

- Facilitating Early Stage Researchers (ESR) to work with experienced researchers on large projects, such as the FP7 bids, and, in this way, 'learning from the best'. The STMS in particular have been excellent vehicles for achieving this.
- Opening up opportunities to collaborate with a variety of disciplines within Switzerland as well as between Switzerland and other countries, and participation in a new COST Action, through new memberships from researchers from new disciplines.
- Supporting the development of (new) topic areas and research skills in maternity care, such as client-centred care (Luyben *et al*, 2013), migrant women (Balaam *et al*, 2013), organisational culture (Frith *et al*, 2014) and salutogenesis (Meier Magistretti & Downe *et al*, 2014), and being acknowledged for this. Finally it has facilitated publishing in international peer-reviewed journals, in collaboration with experienced researchers.
- Engagement and development of female researchers and ESR scientists over the life of the Action.
- Developing of associated spin-off projects and collaboration (for example; EU projects, such as Optibirth).
- Engagement in, and developing knowledge about, multiple new social media for both networking and marketing.
- Facilitating a growing national interest in the value of consumers' views and opinions for assessing and improving the quality of maternity care. The results of the studies that have been carried out in this regard have been heartily welcomed by both professional and consumer groups. This is inducing new ways of thinking about optimal maternity care through the perspective of salutogenesis and complexity.

Establishing effective collaborations, both nationally as well as internationally, has been challenging and needed time. A number of challenges had to be faced, firstly in bringing together partners from federalist, highly autonomous, political structures and, secondly, in establishing collaboration between young research disciplines and institutions with highly competitive characters. However, the formal processes and requirements for the position of being a MC member from COST Switzerland, as well as the annual reports, have been structures pushing ongoing efforts for collaboration. Thirdly, dealing with a challenging financial climate has made it hard to find funding for projects. On top of this, time constraints posed on individual researchers due to other obligations also affected achievement of the results of the Action. In addition, the unfavourable exchange rate of the Swiss franc, and thus the high costs of staying in Switzerland, were a barrier to several incoming STS Missions.

In conclusion, our participation in the COST Action has been a good, positive experience. It has established maternity care research in Switzerland as well as positioning Swiss maternity care in the larger European context. A positive effect of some of the 'negative' aspects in Switzerland has meant that there has been a growing need for an interdisciplinary discussion and collaboration, both between professionals and consumers. As a result, there has been increased interest in a Swiss network aiming to improve maternity care.

This chapter is based on the presentation: *Luyben A, Meier Magistretti C, Maffi I, Hurni D, Fink S & Kuhn A (2014). 'Getting Europe into Switzerland and Switzerland into Europe' – Swiss participation in COST Action IS0907. Optimising Childbirth Across Europe, 9-10 April 2014, Brussels.*

Acknowledgements

The authors would like to acknowledge the many persons and institutions that contributed to the results of Action in Switzerland. These are:

Network of institutions within Switzerland with finished or ongoing projects during the period of the COST Action IS0907 and related to the topic: University of Lausanne, Bern University of Applied Sciences (Health Section (Institute of Midwifery) (BFH), Business Section), Lucerne University of Applied Sciences and Arts (HSLU), Zürich University of Applied Sciences

(Institute of Midwifery). University of Applied Sciences of Western Switzerland (Lausanne, Midwifery Programme) (HESAV), University of Applied Sciences of Western Switzerland (Geneva, Midwifery Programme) (HES-SO), University of Basle, University of Bern, University Hospital (Women's Clinic) Bern, Spital STS AG Thun (Women's Clinic), University Hospital of Geneva (Women's Clinic), University Hospital of Lausanne (Women's Clinic), University Hospital Zürich (Women's Clinic).

Collaborations of these institutions and researchers as a result of the Action: University of Central Lancashire, Preston (UK), University of Liverpool (UK), Bournemouth University (UK), University of Ulster (UK), Yale University (USA), University of Norwich (UK), University of Göteborg (Sweden), Vestfold University College Tønsberg (Norway), Hannover Medical School (Germany), University of Liverpool (UK), University of Osnabrück (Germany), North-West University (South Africa), University of Applied Sciences, Innsbruck (Austria).

Furthermore, we want to acknowledge multiple persons and institutions, who contributed to our results, such as Gynécologie Suisse (SGGG), the Schweizerischer Hebammenverband (SHV), Swiss Paediatrics, Schweizerischer Fachverband Mütter- und Väterberatung, Andreas Spichiger, Isabelle Pompizi, Michelle Pichon, Peter Diebold, Luigi Raio, Bruno Guggisberg, Carla Jordi, Thomas Hodel, Dominic Hurni, Patrick Hohlfeld, Daniel Surbek, Iréne Hösli, Roland Zimmermann, Ursula Böhme, Suzanne Grylka, Alexandra Schmidlin, Michel Boulvain, Ruth Erhard, Isabelle Romano, Stefan Fink, Jürgen Stremlow, Rita Bieri, Luzia Häfliger, Dorothée Eichenberger, Simone Villiger, Inez Varga, Patricia Perrenoud, Cornelia Oertle, Karin Messikommer, Elisabeth Zemp, Irène Simmen, Ruth Niederreiter, Ruth Forster Fink, Kirstin Hähnlein, Ilse Steininger, Sue Brailey, Katharina Tritten Schwarz, Rita Herzog, Adrienne Surbek, Brigitte Holzgreve, Ruth-Nunzia Preisig, Barbara Stocker, Michael Lehmann, Urs Sauter, Marianne Haueter, Verena Piguet, Elisabeth Kurth, Madeleine Grüninger, Ingrid Portner, Sascha Hugentobler, Nicola Low, Claudine Burton-Jeangros, Nicole Schmid, Christiane Sutter, Michèlle Pichon, Nadine Oberhauser, Valerie Fleming, and so many others. Thank you.

References

AngloInfo (2015). Health care system in Switzerland. Geneva: AngloInfo. Available from: http://geneva.angloinfo.com/information/healthcare/health-system

Balaam MC, Akerjordet K, Lyberg A, Kaiser B, Schoening E, Fredriksen AM, Ensel A, Gouni IO & Severinsson E (2013). A qualitative review of migrant women's perceptions of their needs and experiences related to pregnancy and childbirth. *J Adv Nurs* 69(9):1919-1930.

Burkhardt K, Forster Fink R & Luyben A (2013). MatHER-ch.ch: Geburtserfahrungen von Frauen in drei Schweizer Kantonen. *Hebamme.ch* 111(4): 4-8.

Chalmers B, Dzakpasu S, Heaman M & Kaczorowski J for the Maternity Care Experiences Study Group (2008). The Canadian Maternity Experiences Survey: an overview of findings. *J Obstet Gynaecol Can* 30(3): 217-228.

De Graeve D, Hermann I, Kesteloot K, Jegers M & Gilles W (2001). Zwitserland. *Acta Hospitalia* 1: 85-95.

DeVries R, Benoit C, Van Teijlingen ER & Wrede S (2001). *Birth by Design*. New York: Routledge.

Downe S (2009). Memorandum of Understanding COST Action ISCH 0907. Childbirth cultures, concerns and consequences: Creating a dynamic EU framework for optimal maternity care. Available from: www.cost.eu/COST_Actions/isch/Actions/IS0907

Esmail N (2013). *Health Care Lessons from Switzerland: Lessons from Abroad*. A series on health care reform. Vancouver: Fraser Institute. Available from: www.fraserinstitute.org

European Observatory on Health Care Systems (2000). *Health Care Systems in Transition*. Switzerland. Copenhagen: WHO Regional Office for Europe.

Frith L, Sinclair M, Vehviläinen-Julkunen K, Beeckman K, Loytved C & Luyben A (2014). Organisational culture in midwifery care: a scoping review. *Evidence Based Midwifery* 12, 1 (March), 16-22. Available from: www.rcm.org.uk/ebm/volume-12-2014/volume-12-issue-1/organisational-culture-in-maternity-care-a-scoping-review

Gillen P, Brailey S & Luyben A (2012). Erfahrungen von Hebammen mit Mobbing während ihrer Ausbildung [Experiences of midwives with mobbing during their education]. Poster presentation, Schweizer Hebammenkongress "Selbstbewusste Hebamme, Selbstbewusste Frau" [Swiss Midwives' Congress "Confident midwife, Confident woman"], Schwyz, Switzerland, 23/24 May 2012.

Luyben AG & Gross MM (2001). Intrapartum fetal heart rate monitoring: do Swiss midwives implement evidence into practice? *Eur J Obstet Gynecol Reprod Biol* 96(2):179-182.

Luyben A (2011). Europäisches Forschungsprojekt zur bestmöglichen Betreuung während der Schwangerschaft [European research project to provide optimal care during pregnancy]. Hebamme.ch 109: 7-8, 37-38.

Luyben A, Burkhardt K, Conca A, Gurtner-Zürcher C, Hähnlein K, Brailey S & Forster Fink R (2013). MatHER-ch.ch: Maternal Health Experiences Research during Childbirth in Switzerland. Wirksamkeit der Betreuung auf die Gesundheit rund um die Geburt aus Sicht der Frauen in drei Schweizer Kantonen (Studie GFY-5.0007.01). Schlussbericht. Bern: Berner Fachhochschule.

Luyben A (2010). Europäisches Forschungsprojekt zur bestmöglichen Betreuung während der Schwangerschaft [European research project to provide optimal care during pregnancy]. *Frequenz, Das Magazin des Fachbereichs Gesundheit der Berner Fachhochschule*. Dezember: 18-19.

Luyben A, Forster Fink R, Brailey S, Fink S & Van Teijlingen E (2014). MatHER-ch.ch: Piloting the Maternal Experiences Survey (MES) questionnaire for surveying women's experiences of maternity care in Switzerland. Optimising Childbirth Across Europe, 9-10 April 2014, Brussels.

Luyben A, Kaiser B, Meier Magistretti C, Kuhn A (2011). Creating an optimal framework for maternity care – Swiss participation in COST Action IS0907 'Childbirth Culture, Concerns and Consequences'. Poster. 'Zeit für...', Schweizer Hebammenkongress, Fribourg, 12/13 May 2011.

Luyben JG (2008). Mothering the mother. A study of effective content of care during pregnancy from women's points of view in three European countries. Doctoral thesis. Glasgow: Caledonian University.

Maffi I (2013). Can caesarean section be 'natural'? The hybrid nature of the nature-culture dichotomy in mainstream obstetric culture. *Journal for Research in Sickness and Society 10*, 19: 5-26.

Meier Magistretti C, Downe S, Tritten Schwarz K, Berg M, Lindström B (2014). Best practice in maternity care: a salutogenic approach. Optimising Childbirth Across Europe, 9-10 April 2014, Brüssels.

Meier Magistretti C, Rabhi-Sidler S, Villiger S, Luyben A, Auerbach S, Varga I (2014). Wenn die Geburt der Tod ist: Nachgeburtliche Betreuung bei perinatalem Kindstod [If birth is death: postnatal care after perinatal death]. Oktober 2014, Lucerne University of Applied Sciences and Arts/ Hochschule Luzern. Available from: www.hslu.ch/s-pug-projekte

Meier Magistretti C, Villiger S, Luyben A, Varga I (2013). Qualität und Lücken in der postnatalen Betreuung [Quality and gaps in postnatal care]. March 2013, Lucerne University of Applied Sciences and Arts. Available from: http://www.hslu.ch/s-projektbericht_postnatalcare.pdf

Newburn M, Bhavnani V (2010). *Left to your own devices: the postnatal experiences of 1260 first-time mothers*. London: National Childbirth Trust. Available from: www.nct.org.uk/sites/default/files/related_documents/PostnatalCareSurveyReport5.pdf

Organisation for Economic Cooperation and Development and World Health Organization (OECD/WHO) (2011). *OECD Reviews of Health Systems: Switzerland 2011*. Paris: OECD.

Oertle Bürki C (2008). Fachhochschulen Gesundheit in der Schweiz. Konzeption und Aufbau im Umfeld der allgemeinen Fachhochschulentwicklung [Universities of Applied Sciences for Health in Switzerland. Concept and development in the general context of the development of the Universities of Applied Sciences]. Bern: Peter Lang.

Swiss Federal Statistical Office SFSO (2013). Swiss average overall with few exceptions. 2010 European Perinatal Health Report. Press Release. Bern: SFSO Available from: www.news.admin.ch/message/index.html?lang=en&msg-id=48963

Swiss Federal Statistical Office SFSO (2015). Statistisches Lexikon der Schweiz. Bevölkerungsdaten im Vergleich. Bern: SFSO. Available from: www.bfs.admin.ch/bfs/portal/de/index/themen/01.html

Schweizerischer Hebammenverband SHV (2014). Personal mail information Chr. Rieben.

White J, Schouten M, Berg M, Meier Magistrettti M (2014). Stakeholder engagement and the diffusion of childbirth knowledge: experiences of the COST project. Optimising Childbirth Across Europe, 9-10 April 2014, Brüssels.

Zeitlin J, Mohangoo A & Delnord M (2010). *European Perinatal Health Report: Health and Care of Pregnant Women and Babies in 2010*. Paris: Euro-Peristat. Available from: www.europeristat.com/images/doc/Peristat%202013%20V2.pdf

CHAPTER 10

Technology in childbirth: exploring women's views of fetal monitoring during labour – a systematic review

Valerie Smith, Cecily Begley and Declan Devane

Introduction

In evaluating and implementing healthcare interventions, the perspectives and experiences of the individuals directly concerned with those interventions are important. This applies when interventions appear to be beneficial, as well as when evidence suggests they are harmful, or when the evidence base is not strong enough to resolve uncertainty. The findings of previous research demonstrate that there is a lack of supporting evidence for admission cardiotocography (ACTG) and continuous electronic fetal monitoring (EFM) during labour, when compared to intermittent auscultation (IA) of the fetal heart rate (FHR), in low-risk women (Devane *et al*, 2012; Alfirevic *et al*, 2013). Yet, the use of ACTG and EFM in low-risk women remains widespread (Kaczorowski *et al*, 1998; Devane *et al*, 2007; Holzmann & Nordstrom, 2010).

The perspective of women can provide important insights and understandings on the use and choice of FHR monitoring methods. In addition, such perspectives may offer some explanation for continuing with practices that are contrary to current evidence. In this chapter, we explore FHR monitoring technology from the perspectives and experience of women as a group of individuals affected directly by the application of FHR monitoring during labour.

Aim

The aim of this systematic review is to offer insight and understanding, through summary, aggregation and interpretation of findings from studies reporting women's views, experiences or perspectives on FHR monitoring during labour.

Methods

Systematic reviews have focused traditionally on studies evaluating the effects of healthcare interventions and are thus frequently limited to reports of randomised and quasi-randomised trials, with pooling and statistical analysis (meta-analysis) of study results where appropriate (Goldsmith *et al*, 2007). Increasingly, however, consideration is being given to synthesising the findings from qualitative enquiries, with many examples of such syntheses now available in the literature (O'Connell & Downe, 2007; Lundgren *et al*, 2012; Smith *et al*, 2012). An important benefit of this type of synthesis is in the potential to identify particular views, experiences, priorities and concerns not readily identified by systematic reviews of quantitative studies. The evidence from qualitative research, either on its own or incorporated into the findings of systematic reviews of intervention studies, may assist the successful implementation of effective interventions and may have implications for the identification of remaining uncertainties and the need for future research (Dixon-Woods *et al*, 2001; Dixon-Woods *et al*, 2006; Goldsmith *et al*, 2007).

In addition to using traditional qualitative methods such as interviews, studies exploring women's perspectives or experiences might also use more quantitative-orientated methods, such as questionnaires and surveys. A thorough review of the literature, in addition to consulting experts in the field of data synthesis, was performed to identify a framework or an established approach for summarising evidence of this type. Of particular interest was a report by Thomas and colleagues (Thomas *et al*, 2003) from the Evidence for Policy and Practice Information and Coordinating (EPPI) Centre, at the Institute of Education in London, England. One of the two reviews contained in their report details a synthesis of children's views on healthy eating that included both qualitative and quantitative studies. The framework used in this review provided a guide to our review of women's views of FHR monitoring during labour.

Search and selection strategy

The electronic databases of MEDLINE (1966-May 2015), CINAHL (1986-May 2015), EMBASE (1974-May 2015) and Maternity and Infant Care: MIDIRS (1971-May 2015) were searched. Search terms used to guide the search included; *'fetal monitoring'*, *'fetal monitor'*, *'fetal assessment'*, *'cardiotocography'*, *'pregnancy'*, *'childbirth'*, *'perceptions'*, *'views'* and *'experiences'*. These were combined using the Boolean operands 'OR' and 'AND' as appropriate (Table 1 provides an example). Papers were screened initially by title and by abstract, and full texts were retrieved for those citations considered potentially relevant for inclusion. Reference lists of retrieved full text papers were examined to identify potentially relevant studies not captured by the electronic search (Horsley *et al*, 2011). Searches were limited to English language publications because of unavailability of funding for language translation.

Table 1:
Sample search strategy

#	CINAHL: MAY 11 2015	RESULTS
S4	S1 AND S2 AND S3	104
S3	qualitative/ti.ab OR perceptions/ti.ab OR perception/ti.ab OR experiences/ti.ab OR experience/ti.ab OR views/ti.ab	169,032
S2	intermittent auscultation/ti.ab OR cardiotocograph/ti.ab OR cardiotocography/ti.ab OR CTG/ti.ab OR fetal assessment/ti.ab OR fetal monitor/ti.ab OR fetal monitoring/ti.ab	837
S1	EXP/Pregnancy OR EXP/Childbirth OR antenatal/kw. OR prenatal/kw. OR labour/kw. OR ante-natal/kw. OR ante-partum/kw. OR intrapartum/kw. OR intra-partum/kw.	113,271

ti.ab: title and abstract; kw: key word; EXP/: major subject heading term exploded

Inclusion/exclusion criteria

The PEOS (participants/exposure/outcomes/study type) acronym was used to determine the review's inclusion criteria and to guide the selection of studies to answer the review aim (Table 2).

Table 2:
Inclusion criteria

CRITERION	DESCRIPTION
Participants	Pregnant or postpartum women
Exposure	Any method of FHR monitoring during labour
Outcomes	Views, experiences or attitudes towards any method of FHR monitoring during labour
Study type	All studies, irrespective of study design, whose specific aim was to explore and report on women's views, perspectives or experiences towards any method of FHR monitoring during labour*

** This did not include studies that aimed broadly to explore women's experiences of labour and birth, recognising, at the same time, that data related to FHR monitoring might be available in such studies. This decision was consciously made to ensure a clearly defined review scope and to ensure depth, rather than breadth, of data in addressing the review aim.*

Quality assessment

In line with standard systematic review methodology we performed a formal methodological quality appraisal of each included study. The 12 criteria, developed by the EPPI-Centre for their review on healthy eating in young children (Thomas *et al*, 2003) were used to guide this assessment (Table 3).

Data extraction

Data extraction required a careful line-by-line review, immersion in the study, and a breakdown of each included study's findings. Although labour intensive, this process was essential because the reports on the included studies varied in writing styles and publication formats. By deconstructing the findings of each study carefully, we were able to determine and retrieve the relevant data to meet the aim of our review. Data extraction tables (Tables 4, 5 and 6) were designed and predetermined prior to the data extraction process. These tables allowed us to present each study in a standard format and made it easier to compare and contrast between studies, and summary aspects of the review.

Table 3:

EPPI-Centre quality appraisal criteria

CRITERION	DESCRIPTION
Quality of study reporting	
A	Aims and objectives were clearly reported
B	Adequate description of context of research
C	Adequate description of the sample and sampling methods
D	Adequate description of data collection methods
E	Adequate description of data analysis methods
There was some or a good attempt to establish:	
F	Reliability of data collection tools
G	Validity of data collection tools
H	Reliability of data analysis
I	Validity of data analysis
Quality of methods	
J	Used appropriate data collection methods to allow for expression of views
K	Used appropriate methods for ensuring the analysis was grounded in the views
L	Actively involved participants in the design and conduct of the study

Data analysis

A thematic analysis of the findings of each included study was performed. Thematic analysis involves the identification of prominent or recurrent themes in the literature and the synthesis of findings from studies under thematic headings. It has been described as flexible, allowing considerable latitude to reviewers, and is a means of integrating qualitative and quantitative evidence (Horsley *et al*, 2011).

The steps used to conduct the thematic analysis were adopted from Lucas *et al* (2007) and involved the following:

1. Data were extracted from the included studies' findings and entered into a table for later consideration (Table 6);
2. When ready to consider the findings of each study, we referred to the data in Table 6 and identified emergent themes from the individual study's findings;

3. A list of themes was produced for each study (last column of Table 6). The relevant section of the findings related to the particular identified theme was highlighted (bold font) to clarify the association between the findings and the list of themes (Table 6);
4. A synthesis of the findings was performed. Data synthesis was iterative and involved going back and forth between the original papers and the data extraction tables.

Results

Search and selection strategy

The search strategy identified a total of 166 citations of which 149 were excluded at title/abstract screening because they were not about women's views of FHR monitoring during labour. This left 17 citations for full text review after which seven were excluded for the following reasons: one was a narrative review on the responses of women to FHR monitoring (Syndal, 1988), one was a duplicate publication (Starkman, 1977), one explored women's views on decision-making and was not explicitly about monitoring the FHR (Davey *et al*, 2004), and four (Jackson *et al*, 1983; Hansen *et al*, 1985; Shalev *et al*, 1985; Killien & Shy, 1989) were either non-comparable in design with the included studies or were not reported in a way that allowed us to extract and present themes from the data. For example, Shalev *et al* (1985) reported on maternal biochemical responses to EFM as measured by blood stress-hormone levels and Killien & Shy (1989) reported group differences on items using mean scores and standard deviations.

A total of ten papers (Dulock & Herron, 1976; Starkman, 1976; Shields, 1978; Beck, 1980; McDonough *et al*, 1981; Hodnett, 1982; Molfese *et al*, 1982; Garcia *et al*, 1985; Hindley *et al*, 2008; Barber *et al*, 2013) including 677 participants, were thus included in the review. Details of the characteristics of included studies are provided in Tables 4 and 5. Figure 1 provides a flow diagram of the search and selection strategy.

Figure 1:
Search and selection flow diagram (Moher *et al*, 2009)

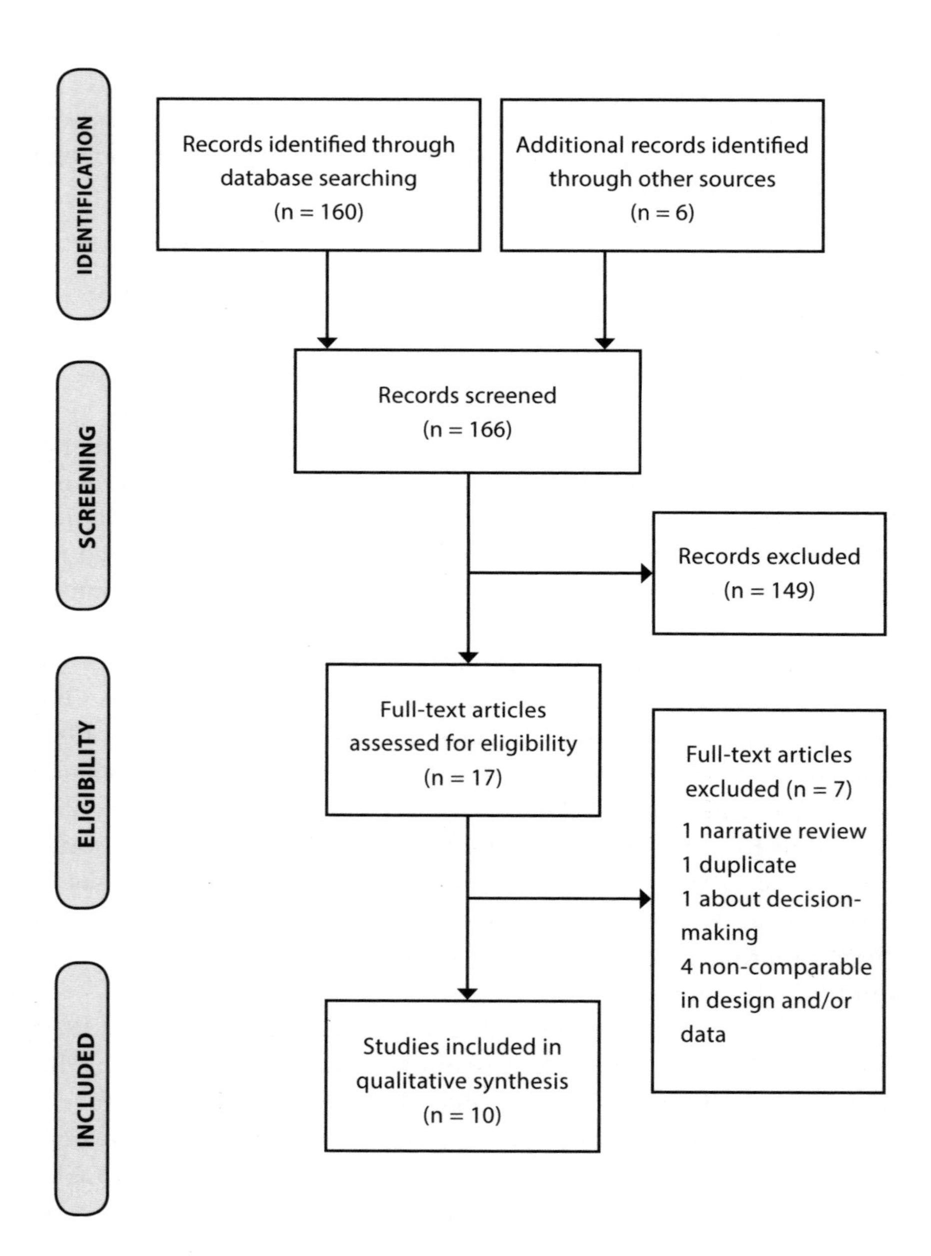

Table 4:

Summary of descriptive characteristics of included studies

STUDY	AIM	STUDY LOCATION	PARTICIPANTS	TIMING
Dulock & Herron	To investigate if monitoring during labour adversely affects the childbirth experience	Moffitt Hospital, San Francisco	31 women	2-3 days post-birth
Starkman	To gain insight into the psychological effects of EFM	University Medical Centre, USA	25 women	Post-birth while still in hospital
Shields	To explore women's reactions to internal EFM	USA	30 women	Within 48 hours of birth
Beck	To investigate women's reactions to fetal monitoring	350-bedded maternity unit, Baltimore, USA	50 women	3 days post-birth
McDonough	To understand parents' reactions to the fetal monitor	Bethesda Hospital, USA	50 women	1 day post-birth
Hodnett	To investigate the effects of two types of monitoring (standard or radiotelemetric EFM) in labour on ability to maintain control during labour	Toronto, Canada	30 women	Within 48 hours of birth
Molfese	To examine reactions to intrapartum fetal monitoring	University Hospital and Community Hospital, USA	180 women	1-2 days post-birth
Garcia	To explore views related to method of FHR monitoring (IA and CTG)	Dublin, Ireland	200 women	Post-birth while still in hospital
Hindley	To ascertain women's views on intrapartum fetal monitoring techniques	Two units, England	63 AN 38/63 PN	-
Barber	To investigate whether the use of EFM during labour increases or reduces anxiety levels among women	Two centres in the UK taking part in the INFANT Study	18 women	-

Table 5:

Summary of methodological characteristics of included studies

STUDY	SAMPLING METHODS	DATA COLLECTION	DATA ANALYSIS
Dulock & Herron	Non-probability sample	Questionnaire and interviews	Descriptive; frequencies
Starkman	Non-probability sample	Interviews – structured and responses scored	Descriptive, Fisher Exact Probabilities test, Student's t-test
Shields	Non-probability sample	Interviews and 'Moods & Feelings Inventory' to ascertain positive and negative attitudes	Inventory scores, Chi-square
Beck	Non-probability sample	Interviews	Descriptive, Chi-square
McDonough	Non-probability sample	Questionnaire and interviews	Descriptive; counts and comments
Hodnett	Random sampling	Questionnaire; 'Labour Agentry Scale' and interviews	Student's t-test, Fisher's exact test, Chi-squared test
Molfese	Random sampling	Questionnaire and interviews	Descriptive; mean, standard deviation, Factor analysis
Garcia	Random sampling	Semi-structured questionnaire	Frequencies, Chi-square, t-test
Hindley	Non-probability sampling	Questionnaire (survey research)	Descriptive; frequency counts, cross-tabulations
Barber	Non-probability sampling	Visual analogue scale (1-10) for anxiety and interviews	ANCOVA; thematic analysis

Table 6:

Data extraction

STUDY	KEY FINDINGS REPORTED BY AUTHORS OF STUDY *(sample data only provided for illustrative purposes)*	EMERGING THEMES
Dulock & Herron	77% (24/31) – positive comments; **seeing the contraction on the printout** helped them control their breathing and relaxation; 90% (28/31) commented positively about being able to hear the FHR from the monitor – related almost always to feelings of safety and security; many women also stated that being on the monitor increased their husbands' **feelings of security in relation to fetal wellbeing**; 70% (22/31) had some negative comments about EFM, mainly associated with the external belts; **'too tight'**, **'feelings of confinement'**, **'lack of mobility'** and 'interference with abdominal massage'; one woman stated that being on the monitor made her **feel nervous.**	Information Reassurance Safety Mobility Discomfort Anxiety/Fear
Starkman	The fetal monitor as: 1) **Protector** – **reassured in the presence of the monitor;** protecting against disaster – **guaranteeing the baby would survive**; 2) Extension of patient v **providing information on their labour** to the doctor; 3) Aid in **communication** – **communicated for and about them,** making it easier for them to initiate conversation with their doctor; 4) Extension of baby – hearing the FHR **confirmed baby was alive**; 5) Affecting interactions with husband – **facilitated participation of husbands** in the experience of labour; 6) A distraction – pass time watching the monitor; 7) Aid in mastery – being **alerted that contractions were coming** and able to get ready for their impact; 8) Competitive feelings – staff and husband hovering over/looking at monitor; 9) Mechanical monster – **physical discomfort, enforced immobility,** monitor malfunctions and **fear of sounds** from the monitor; 10) Producing increased **anxiety** – concern about injury to the baby (relates to scalp electrode) and **anxiety** due to noises from the monitor (especially if FHR slowed).	Reassurance Safety Information Communication Discomfort Mobility Anxiety/Fear
Shields	22 women were in the positive scores range, 8 were in the negative range; one woman felt that there was 'too **little information**' about the monitor and associated equipment, but 27/30 women thought they had received enough information; 7 women indicated that they **were reassured by the machine**, and therefore had **no worries**; although 11 **had worries** about the baby during monitoring and one was **'a little frightened'**. The most frequent complaint was **difficulty in getting comfortable; noise of the FHR** was discomforting as they were **fearful that it would stop**; one woman felt that staff had **more interest in the machine** than in her.	Information Anxiety/Fear Reassurance Discomfort Communication

STUDY	KEY FINDINGS REPORTED BY AUTHORS OF STUDY *(sample data only provided for illustrative purposes)*	EMERGING THEMES
Beck	Some initial positive responses; women glad of the monitor so their **husband's could see a contraction** and help them breathe; happy – they could hear that their **babies' heartbeats were strong**; some initial negative reactions included **fear** that the **monitor would cause them 'pain'**; 74% of women had positive subsequent responses; **'a safeguard'** and **'very informative'.** Many women felt secure – **reassuring to hear the heartbeat** – allowed them to relax and **not worry**; Negative subsequent responses mainly centred on the **discomfort caused by the belts** and a **fear that the belts** pressing in would **hurt their babies**; the feeling of **being tied down** which was **frightening.** For one woman, the monitor made her **nervous** and it **made it 'hurt more'.**	Information Communication Anxiety/Fear Safety Reassurance Discomfort Mobility
McDonough	Mother's reported that they were **not fearful** for their babies during labour **because the monitor** was being used (47/50); one mother thought her baby might have **died but for the monitor**, although some mothers were concerned that the **internal monitor might 'hurt'** their baby; 44/50 did not report **discomfort due to the monitor**, 47/50 felt **less fear** with the monitor; 49/50 did not think the nurse was **more interested in the monitor** than in her; only 5/50 reported that the monitor made them **nervous.**	Reassurance Safety Anxiety/Fear Discomfort Communication
Hodnett	9/15 in the standard EFM group **did not get out of bed at all during labour**; all 15 in the radiotelemetric group, **which allows women to ambulate**, spent some time out of bed. 28 of the 30 participants (14 from each group) stated that the monitor had an effect on their labour experiences. The responses varied across groups; those receiving radiotelemetric monitoring **were reassured as to the condition** of the fetus and **felt freedom from restraint;** those receiving standard EFM described negative effects including **discomfort associated with the abdominal belts, interference with movement and comfort,** especially during contractions and that the monitor made them **anxious.**	Mobility Reassurance Discomfort Anxiety/Fear
Molfese	The monitor as a **protector of the baby,** the monitor as an understandable **source of information** for staff and women; they were able to use the information from the monitor in a variety of ways – contraction mastery, involvement of husband in the birth process and **reassurance about baby's wellbeing**; strong agreements from women the **monitor was there to help** and **staff were knowledgeable** about the equipment; women disagreed that the monitor **provided little information** for the doctor, that staff paid more attention to it than to women or that it was distressing or annoying; there were aspects of the monitor that women did not like – some felt the **straps uncomfortable** and **equipment breakdowns worried** or annoyed them.	Safety Information Reassurance Communication Discomfort Anxiety/Fear

STUDY	KEY FINDINGS REPORTED BY AUTHORS OF STUDY *(sample data only provided for illustrative purposes)*	EMERGING THEMES
Garcia	Women monitored by standard EFM felt more **restricted in their movements;** one woman described **discomfort caused by the monitor belt;** the data did not support the premise that staff attention might be divided between the monitor and women, although women who received EFM were more often **left alone** for short periods and many of them did mind this (35/55); EFM was not more **reassuring** to mothers than IA; for some women (27%) the monitor had broken down at some point during labour and this was **upsetting and frightening** for some women.	Mobility Discomfort Communication Anxiety/Fear
Hindley	Women would prefer to **stay mobile** in labour; however, 40% (n=16/38) reported staying on the bed during labour; more women who had EFM choose epidural compared to women who had IA (53% versus 39%); women wanted to remain **in control** but 38% of women indicated that they had conceded decision-making powers on method of monitoring to midwives during labour; women also indicated that **choice was very important** to them, however, 94% indicated that **midwives did not facilitate choice** in FHR monitoring method. Women relied on multiple sources for **information** including midwives; however 65% (n=41/63) indicated that the **midwife had not explicitly given any information** on FHR monitoring.	Mobility Discomfort Communication Control Choice Information
Barber	Women commonly reported **finding monitoring reassuring** and that it helped **reassure the father too,** and could generate **a sense of involvement** because they could see a contraction coming and support their partner appropriately. Women voiced that being monitored **restricted their movements;** common objections to monitoring were because of **restrictions on freedom of movement.** Women talked about wanting to relieve pain by moving around and how **the monitor inhibited this**. Also comments about it **feeling uncomfortable** and **anxiety** increased for women with the urgent comments and behaviour of staff as they **responded to the monitoring results**; one woman spoke of how **everyone was focused on the monitor** and this was causing her **stress.**	Reassurance Mobility Discomfort Anxiety/Fear Communication

Quality assessment

Table 7 details the results of the quality assessment of the studies included in the review. None of the included studies reported on all 12 criteria in their papers. One study (Molfese *et al,* 1982) addressed 11 of the 12 criteria in their paper, and one study (Barber *et al,* 2013) addressed 10 of the 12 criteria. Shields (1978) scored the lowest on quality assessment, addressing only three of the 12 criteria, while Dulock & Herron (1976) and McDonough *et al* (1981) scored the second lowest, addressing only four of the 12 quality assessment criteria.

Table 7:

Results of quality appraisal of included studies

STUDY	QUALITY CRITERIA MET
Dulock & Herron	A, B, C, J
Starkman	A, B, C, D, E, F, H, J, K
Shields	A, D, E
Beck	B, C, D, E
McDonough	A, B, C, J
Hodnett	A, B, C, D, E, F, J, K
Molfese	A, B, C, D, E, F, G, H, I, J, K
Garcia	A, B, C, D, E, F, H, J, K
Hindley	A, B, C, D, E, F, G, J, K
Barber	A, B, C, D, E, F, G, H, I, J

Thematic analysis

Table 8 provides an overview of the emergent themes from each of the ten included studies. From these, four dominant themes were identified and subjected to thematic analysis to present a comprehensive synthesis of women's views of FHR monitoring in practice. These themes were 1) discomfort, 2) anxiety / fear, 3) reassurance, and 4) communication. Some of the other emergent themes were identified as sub-themes of dominant themes and were explored and analysed as such. For example, safety was closely associated with reassurance. Mobility, or more specifically, immobility, was often associated with discomfort due to an inability to freely move as a direct result of being connected to the FHR monitor.

Table 8:

Overview of emerging themes from included studies

THEME/STUDY	1	2	3	4	5	6	7	8	9	10
Communication	x	x	x	x	x	-	x	x	x	x
Information	-	x	x	x	-	-	x	-	x	-
Reassurance	x	x	x	x	x	x	x	-	-	x
Safety	x	x	-	x	x	-	x	-	-	-
Mobility	x	x	-	x	-	x	-	x	x	x
Discomfort	x	x	x	x	x	x	x	x	x	x
Anxiety/Fear	x	x	x	x	x	x	x	x	-	x
Control	-	-	-	-	-	-	-	-	x	-
Choice	-	-	-	-	-	-	-	-	x	-

1. Discomfort

Discomfort emerged as a theme in all ten of the included studies and was associated strongly with discomfort from EFM equipment such as the internal fetal scalp electrode or the abdominal transducer and belts, which were often described as too tight and contributed to increased pain (Dulock & Herron, 1976; Beck, 1980):

> *'I was nervous. I didn't like the machine at all. It made it hurt more'* (Beck, 1980: 352).

Women also reported discomfort arising from enforced immobility associated with EFM and considerable restrictions on freedom of movement (Dulock & Herron, 1976; Starkman, 1976; Beck, 1980; Hodnett, 1982; Garcia *et al*, 1985; Barber *et al*, 2013), which contrasted with their wishes to remain mobile (Hindley *et al*, 2008):

> *'...I felt tied down and couldn't get out of bed. I felt like Frankenstein's bride'* (Beck, 1980: 352).

The view that EFM restricted movement was significant in the Garcia *et al* (1985) study with 17% (n=17) of women in the EFM group compared with

6% (n=6) in the IA group ($p < 0.05$) reporting that freedom of movement was too restricted. EFM also appeared to increase the need for analgesia. In one study, women who received IA during labour (n=15) did not request epidural analgesia; however, all women who received continuous EFM during labour (n=20) had either an epidural or a narcotic analgesia (Hindley *et al*, 2008).

Conflicting views in relation to the degree of discomfort experienced by women, depending on the method of FHR monitoring used, were also evident. For example, when comparing IA with EFM, women reported that:

> *'The machine is probably more comfortable than the fetal stethoscope pressing on your tummy'* (Garcia *et al*, 1985: 83).

Women expressed a preference for the fetal monitor because:

> *'it was uncomfortable for me to keep turning on my back for the nurse to listen in to the baby'* (Garcia *et al*, 1985: 83).

Similarly, when comparing radiotelemetric monitoring, which allows women to ambulate, with EFM by standard CTG, women in the radiotelemetric monitoring group experienced greater freedom from restraint. Contrastingly, women who were monitored by standard CTG described interference with movement and comfort (Molfese *et al*, 1982). For some women, however, any method of FHR monitoring caused a certain degree of discomfort:

> *'Towards the end of labour I found both the belts and the nurses listening in very uncomfortable'* (Garcia *et al*, 1985: 83).

2. Anxiety / fear

The theme of anxiety and fear emerged in nine of the ten included studies (Starkman, 1976; Shields, 1978; Beck, 1980; McDonough *et al*, 1981; Hodnett, 1982; Molfese *et al*, 1982; Garcia *et al*, 1985; Hindley *et al*, 2008; Barber *et al*, 2013). The experience of anxiety and/or fear was, in the main, associated with the auditory sounds emitted from the monitor. Women became frightened when the monitor alarmed, as would happen if the transducer or internal scalp electrode became detached (Starkman, 1976; Beck, 1980;

Molfese *et al*, 1982). In addition, hearing the baby's heartbeat evoked fear and anxiety for some women, particularly if the baby's heartbeat slowed at any point during labour (Starkman, 1976; Shields, 1978; Beck, 1980):

> *'Then the monitor started to show the fetal heart rate go down. It was so hard for my husband to see and hear it that he had to leave the room'* (Starkman, 1976: 273).

> *'When the machine first started to beep, the baby's heartbeat was so fast that I thought he was in cardiac arrest'* (Beck, 1980: 352).

Electronic fetal monitoring equipment itself evoked fear and anxiety in some women. Many were concerned that the equipment might hurt either them or their baby:

> *'I thought I was going to be electrocuted. My water had broke. The cord of the machine was lying in the water'* (Beck, 1980: 351).

One woman was:

> *'worried the whole time that the baby's heart would stop if the machine stopped'* (Shields, 1978: 2112).

Anxiety levels were increased in women who experienced internal EFM. More than one-quarter of the participants in one study expressed concern that the fetal scalp electrode might injure the baby or puncture the 'soft spot' (Shields, 1978):

> *'The head is the most important part and I was worried about brain damage because of the clip'* (Shields, 1978: 2112).

EFM equipment malfunction also caused considerable anxiety for women:

> *'... if the machine breaks down it is frightening'* (Garcia *et al*, 1985: 83).

In Garcia's (1985) study, 27% of the 100 women who had EFM said that the equipment malfunctioned at some point during labour and, of these, one third experienced anxiety and fear because of this.

3. Reassurance

Reassurance emerged as a prominent theme in eight of the ten included studies and was almost always related to hearing the baby's heartbeat (Dulock & Herron, 1976; Starkman, 1976; Shields, 1978; Beck, 1980; McDonough *et al*, 1981; Hodnett, 1982; Molfese *et al*, 1982; Barber *et al*, 2013):

> *'I was happy. This way I hear myself that my baby's heart was strong'* (Beck, 1980: 351).

> *'I did quite enjoy having the monitors on actually…you can just see sort of their heartbeat and how strong your contractions were…'* (Barber *et al*, 2013: 399).

EFM was linked strongly to the notion of safety and security. It was described as a safeguard, reassuring them, and their partners, of the wellbeing of their baby, helping them, in turn to relax and not to worry (Dulock & Herron, 1976; Beck, 1980; Barber *et al*, 2013). For some women, EFM confirmed to them that their baby was still alive (Starkman, 1976; Beck, 1980) and some women considered the monitor as a tool that would ensure the survival of the baby:

> *'…The monitor was watching it, keeping track of it. I knew that at least the baby would live…'* (Starkman, 1976: 272)

Women who had a caesarean section during their labour felt that their baby might have died or been born seriously ill had it not been for the fetal monitor (Beck, 1980; McDonough *et al*, 1981):

> *'The monitor saved my baby's life because the doctor knew to do a caesarean section'* (Beck, 1980: 351).

This view was also held by women who had lost a baby in a previous pregnancy or labour (Starkman, 1976) and by women of lower income when compared to women of upper income levels (Molfese *et al*, 1982).

4. Communication

Communication emerged as a dominant theme in nine of the ten included studies (Dulock & Herron, 1976; Starkman, 1976; Shields, 1978; Beck, 1980; McDonough *et al*, 1981; Molfese *et al*, 1982; Garcia *et al*, 1985; Hindley *et al*, 2008; Barber *et al*, 2013) and was associated strongly with the provision of information:

> *'It was good to see that the contractions were real and not psychological or my own impression. That way the doctor could get real information'* (Starkman, 1976: 272).

The CTG machine was viewed as a focal point for women to initiate conversations with their carers (Starkman, 1976) and, for some women, the use of EFM facilitated the participation of their husbands in the process of childbirth, generating, for them, a sense of involvement:

> *'Now my husband could see when I was having a contraction and help me breathe'* (Beck, 1980: 351).

In contrast, some women considered EFM a hindrance to effective communication between them and their carers (Starkman, 1976; Shields, 1978; Molfese *et al*, 1982). In such circumstances, EFM diverted attention away from the labouring woman, as clinical staff and birthing partners were perceived to become preoccupied with the monitor:

> *'They all came with the machine and left with the machine'* (Shields, 1978: 2112).

> *'Everyone was just focused on this monitor and the heartbeat, so I think that got a little bit stressful, because I did end up telling him "stop telling me what's happening or talking about it" because it was making me panic'* (Barber *et al*, 2013: 401).

This opinion was also evident in Garcia's (1985) study and, although women in either group did not report feeling less supported, women in the EFM group reported being left alone more often than those women who received IA.

Women considered EFM a valuable source of information for them and for midwives and doctors:

> *'Oh, I thought it was brill, to be honest, because as I say a lot of the time I felt a little bit out of the loop. From where I was sitting I could see all the screens and what was going on'* (Barber *et al*, 2013: 399).

Women perceived that the CTG machine could tell them, and their care-giver, when a contraction was coming in situations of regional analgesia (Dulock & Herron, 1976; Starkman, 1976). Women, midwives and doctors also used it as a tool for the diagnosis of labour (Starkman, 1976; Shields, 1978; McDonough *et al*, 1981):

> *'I was sure I was in labor, but the doctors didn't think so … I was glad the monitor was there to prove that I was really in labor'*
> (Starkman, 1976: 272).

> *'…the monitor says your contractions are mild.'*

to which the woman replied

> *'I'm in labour, not the monitor'* (McDonough *et al*, 1981: 34).

Although women in two studies (Garcia *et al*, 1985; Hindley *et al*, 2008) did not report a preference for one type of monitoring method over another, 94% (n=59/63) of women in the Hindley *et al* (2008) study reported not having a choice on method of FHR monitoring. This demonstrates a lack of communication and information on the benefits and risks of different fetal monitoring methods.

Discussion

This systematic review and thematic analysis has identified themes related to women's views of monitoring the FHR during labour through a synthesis of ten studies on this topic. Four dominant themes were identified as 1) discomfort, 2) anxiety/fear, 3) reassurance and 4) communication.

Women's views of FHR monitoring can influence and affect the routine care received by and offered to women during labour (Walker *et al*, 2001) and can affect their experience of childbirth. Consideration of women's experiences of and perceptions towards FHR monitoring technology is important in understanding this important aspect of care. Despite the finding of this review that EFM caused some women increased anxiety, few studies specifically examine this factor or seek women's opinions. For example, a recent Cochrane Review comparing lactate or pH estimation of fetal blood samples in labour (East *et al*, 2010) found no studies that directly measured maternal satisfaction with fetal monitoring, or anxiety, although one subsequent publication to the Cochrane review was identified that objectively explores anxiety using a 1-10 visual analogue scale in women undergoing two different forms of EFM in a trial (Barber *et al*, 2013).

Contrary to current recommendations (NICE, 2014), the use of EFM in low-risk women remains widespread (Kaczorowski *et al*, 1998; Devane *et al*, 2007; Holzmann & Nordstrom, 2010). This review offers insights into understanding why this might be the case and provides evidence of its effect from the experiences and perspectives of women.

EFM offered some women reassurance because it allowed them to hear their baby's heartbeat, although this experience was frightening for others, especially when they could hear the baby's heartbeat slow down. Discomfort was associated with the use of EFM equipment and due to the reduced mobility associated with fetal monitoring technology. Although use of the fetal stethoscope caused discomfort to some women, it also allowed for increased mobility during labour. A systematic review of controlled trials of maternal positions during labour (Simkin & O'Hara, 2002) demonstrated that women who remained upright (i.e. standing, walking and/or sitting upright) used less narcotic or epidural analgesia, had shorter first stages of labour, and needed less oxytocin to augment labour than women who remained in a supine position, as often occurs when EFM is performed. IA also allowed for close proximity and engagement with women, a view highlighted by women as being important (Garcia *et al*, 1985; Hindley *et al*, 2008). This might facilitate increased communication with women from professionals and ultimately afford professionals a greater view of the overall clinical picture. As Shearer (1979) states:

> *'intrapartum fetal death is not prevented by monitors; it is prevented by an alert doctor [midwife] at the bedside of a labouring woman'* (Shearer, 1979: 127).

All studies included in this review, with the exception of the Hindley *et al* (2008) study and the Barber *et al* (2013) study, were published between the years 1976 and 1985. This is the period when electronic fetal monitors became increasingly available commercially and at a time when continuous fetal monitoring was perceived as providing significant advantages:

> *'...now that the appropriate technology is available the obstetrician may virtually eliminate intrapartum stillbirths and reduce morbidity associated with parturition'* (Filshie, 1974: 36).

Since that time, however, evidence from randomised trials has emerged and has demonstrated a lack of evidence of anticipated benefit for EFM during labour when compared to IA (Devane *et al*, 2012; Alfirevic *et al*, 2013). Although the recent 2008 and 2013 papers did echo many of the views and experiences of women in the earlier studies, it would be worth exploring further as to whether women's views on the topic of FHR monitoring during labour has changed over time, considering especially that EFM use remains widespread and appears culturally, that is within the maternity care environment, acceptable in almost all labours in western societies. In this sense, additional and contemporary research on women's views of fetal monitoring during labour is strongly recommended and urgently needed.

Conclusion

This systematic review and thematic analysis has identified themes related to women's views, perceptions and experiences of FHR monitoring in practice. It has offered insights into some of the reasons for continuous EFM during labour. There is insufficient high-quality evidence demonstrating the impact on clinical outcomes for women and their infants depending on FHR monitoring modality used during labour (Alfirevic *et al*, 2013). Implementing evidence-based care and affecting appropriate practice change regarding FHR monitoring requires consideration of women's views.

This review has identified specific areas for clinical decision-makers to consider when implementing policy and practice change. One such area is the need to educate and inform women on types of FHR monitoring during labour, so that they might make an informed choice on the method of monitoring most suitable to them. Recognising that women can experience fear and discomfort when EFM is applied highlights the need to inform and counsel women on the use of EFM technology. If professionals considered this view, it might also help them to decide to use IA more often for low-risk women. Professionals need to be knowledgeable of the current evidence on EFM if they are to engage in evidence-based care, and regular fetal monitoring education for all staff would provide one opportunity to discuss the views of women, as identified in this review, and form part of the process for effecting evidence-based practice change.

This chapter presents the first systematic review and synthesis of evidence, that the authors are aware of, that considers the views, perceptions and experiences of women on FHR monitoring during labour. It has importance and relevance in advancing systematic review methodology, as it provides an additional example of the synthesis of evidence from both qualitative and quantitative enquiry. Further research is required to establish how some of these views might be addressed (inclusive of psychological and emotional factors), and as to whether these views have considerably changed over time, to ensure the provision and continuation of optimum care for women and their babies.

References

Alfirevic Z, Devane D & Gyte GM (2013). Continuous cardiotocography (CTG) as a form of electronic fetal monitoring (EFM) for fetal assessment during labour. *Cochrane Database of Systematic Reviews* 5: CD006066.

Barber V, Linsell L, Locock L, Powell L, Shakeshaft C, Lean K, Colman J, Juszczak E & Brocklehurst P (2013). Electronic fetal monitoring during labour and anxiety levels in women taking part in a RCT. *Br J Midwifery* 21(6): 394-403.

Beck C (1980). Patient acceptance of fetal monitoring as a helpful tool. *JOGN Nurs* 9(6): 350-353.

Davey H, Lim J, Butow P, Barratt A & Redman S (2007). Women's preferences for and views on decision-making for diagnostic tests. *Soc Sci Med* 58: 1699-1707.

Devane D, Lalor J & Bonnar J (2007). The use of intrapartum electronic fetal heart rate monitoring: a national survey. *Irish Med J* 100(2): 360-362.

Devane D, Lalor J, Daly S, Maguire W & Smith V (2012). Cardiotocography versus intermittent auscultation of fetal heart on admission to labour ward for assessment of fetal wellbeing. *Cochrane Database of Systematic Reviews* 2: CD005122.

Dixon-Woods M, Fitzpatrick R & Roberts K (2001). Including qualitative research in systematic reviews: opportunities and problems. *J Eval Clin Pract* 7(2):125-133.

Dixon-Woods M, Bonas S, Booth A, Jones D, Miller T & Sutton A (2006). How can systematic reviews incorporate qualitative research? A critical perspective. *Qual Health Res* 6(1), 27-44.

Dulock H & Herron M (1976). Women's responses to fetal monitoring. *JOGN Nurs* 5(5 Suppl): 68s-70s.

East CE, Leader LR, Sheehan P, Henshall NE & Colditz PB (2010). Intrapartum fetal scalp lactate sampling for fetal assessment in the presence of a non-reassuring fetal heart trace. *Cochrane Database of Systematic Reviews* 3: CD006174.

Filshie M (1974). Intrapartum fetal monitoring. *Br J Hosp Med* 12: 33-34.

Garcia J, Corry M & MacDonald D (1985). Mother's views of continuous electronic fetal heart monitoring and intermittent auscultation in randomised trials. *Birth* 12(2): 79-86.

Goldsmith M, Bankhead C & Austoker J (2007). Synthesising qualitative and quantitative research in evidence-based patient information. *J Epidemiol Comm Health* 61: 262-270.

Hansen P, Smith S, Neldam S & Osler M (1985). Maternal attitudes to fetal monitoring. *Eur J Obstet Gynecol Reprod Biol* 20: 43-51.

Hindley C, Hinsliff SW & Thomson AM (2008). Pregnant womens' views about choice of intrapartum monitoring of the fetal heart rate: a questionnaire survey. *Int J Nurs Stud* 45(2): 224-231.

Hodnett E (1982). Patient control during labour. Effects of two types of fetal monitors. *JOGN Nurs* 11(2): 94-99.

Holzmann M & Nordstrom L (2010). Follow-up national survey (Sweden) of routines for intrapartum fetal surveillance. *Acta Obstet Gynecol Scand* 89: 712-714.

Horsley T, Dingwall O & Sampson M (2011). Checking reference lists to find additional studies for systematic reviews. *Cochrane Database of Systematic Reviews* 8: MR000026.

Jackson J, Vaughan M, Black P & D'Souza S (1983). Psychological aspects of fetal monitoring: maternal reaction to the position of the monitor and staff behaviour. *J Psychosom Obstet Gynaecol* 2(2): 97-102.

Kaczorowski J, Levitt C, Hanvey L, Avard D & Chance G (1998). A national survey of use of obstetric procedures and technologies in Canadian hospitals: routine or based on existing evidence? *Birth* 25(1): 11-18.

Killien M & Shy K (1989) A randomised trial of electronic fetal monitoring in preterm labour: women's views. *Birth* 16(1): 7-12.

Lucas P, Baird J, Arai L, Law C & Roberts H (2007). Worked examples of alternative methods for the synthesis of qualitative and quantitative research in systematic reviews *BMC Med Res Methodol* 7: 4.

Lundgren I, Begely C, Gross MM & Bondas T (2012). 'Groping through the fog': a metasynthesis of women's experiences on VBAC (vaginal birth after caesarean section). *BMC Pregnancy Childbirth* 12: 85.

McDonough M, Sheriff D & Zimmel P (1981). Parents' responses to fetal monitoring. *MCN Am Journal Matern Child Nurs* 6: 32-34.

Moher D, Liberati A, Tetzlaff J, Altman DG (2009). PRISMA Group: preferred reporting items for systematic reviews and meta-analyses: the PRISMA Statement. BMJ 339: b2535.

Molfese V, Sunshine P & Bennett A (1982). Reactions of women to intrapartum fetal monitoring. *Obstet Gynecol* 59(6): 705-709.

NICE (National Institute of Health and Clinical Excellence) (2014). *Intrapartum Care: Care of Healthy Women and their Babies during Childbirth*. London: RCOG Press.

O'Connell R & Downe S (2009). A metasynthesis of midwives' experiences of hospital practice in publicly funded settings: compliance, resistance and authenticity. *Health* 13: 1-21.

Shalev E, Eran A, Harpaz-Kerpel S & Zuckerman H (1985). Psychogenic stress in women during fetal monitoring (hormonal profile). *Acta Obstet Gynecol Scand* 64: 417-420.

Shearer M (1979). Fetal heart monitoring: for better or for worse? *Compulsory Hospital*, 121:127.

Shields D (1978). Maternal reactions to fetal monitoring. *Am J Nurs* 78(12): 2110-2112.

Simkin O & O'Hara MA (2002). Nonpharmacologic relief of pain during labour: systematic reviews of five methods. *Am J Obstet Gynecol* 186(5 Suppl Nature): s131-s159.

Smith V, Begley C, Clarke M & Devane D (2012). Professionals' views of fetal monitoring during labour: a systematic review and thematic analysis. *BMC Pregnancy Childbirth* 12: 166.

Starkman M (1976). Psychological responses to the use of the fetal monitor during labour. *Pyschosom Med* 38(4): 269-277.

Starkman M (1977). Fetal monitoring: psychologic consequences and management recommendations. *Obstet Gynecol* 50(4): 500-504.

Syndal S (1988). Responses of labouring women to fetal heart rate monitoring: a critical review of the literature. *J Nurse Midwifery* 33(5): 208-216.

Thomas J, Sutcliffe K, Harden A, Oakley A, Oliver S & Rees R (2013). *Children and healthy eating: A systematic review of barriers and facilitators*. London: EPPI-Centre, Institute of Education, University of London.

Walker D, Shunkwiler S & Supanich J (2001). Labor and delivery nurse's attitudes towards intermittent fetal monitoring. *J Midwifery Womens Health* 46(6): 374-380.

CHAPTER 11

Normal birth research: the state of the art, and into the future

Soo Downe

The EU COST Action that was the catalyst for the work presented in this book was set up to *advance scientific knowledge about ways of improving maternity care provision and outcomes by examining what works, for whom, in what circumstances, and by identifying and learning from the best*. The intention was to share, synthesise and extend the work of experts from a range of disciplines, using a common framework of salutogenesis and complexity theory. As the authors in this volume demonstrate, this aim has been achieved. There is, however, still more to do. As the original bid for the COST Action also stated: *bringing all maternity care in Europe up to the standard of the best is the ultimate aim of the European Research Network that will be a result of the Action in the longer term.*

Fulfilment of this intention depends on authentically collaborative working. This moves beyond multidisciplinary conversations. It is dependent on a fusion of disciplinary horizons, to enable new insights that could not result from a simple sharing of ideas. In their concept review, Choi and Pak (2006) align the terms multidisciplinary, interdisciplinary and transdisciplinary working with concepts of being (respectively) additive, interactive, and holistic, noting that these occur on a continuum. Klein provides a more detailed analysis:

> *Interdisciplinary and transdisciplinary research, performance, and evaluation are both generative processes of harvesting, capitalizing, and leveraging multiple expertise. Individual standards must be calibrated, and*

tensions among different disciplinary, professional, and interdisciplinary approaches carefully managed in balancing acts that require negotiation and compromise. Readiness levels are strengthened by antecedent conditions that are flexible enough to allow multiple pathways of integration and collaboration. In both cases, as well, new epistemic communities must be constructed and new cultures of evidence produced. (Klein, 2008 p116)

Building effective transdisciplinary collaboration through the creation of these new epistemic communities and new cultures of evidence entails risks as well as benefits. The risks include fracturing of initial alliances and good intentions through a lack of understanding of the fundamental principles and philosophical frameworks of what the collaboration is trying to do. To an extent, this is an inevitable consequence of bringing together academics whose very disciplinary norms arise from potentially conflicting theoretical perspectives, such as positivism in the STEM (Science, Technology, Engineering and Mathematics) disciplines, and more interpretive/constructionist stances in the social sciences, with the humanities somewhere in between. This scenario could potentially be confounded when those who are collaborating are communicating in a range of languages, that are not only hard to translate literally, but also conceptually.

However, the enormous rewards of persistence in overcoming these complex factors are evident in the chapters in this book, and in the wider outputs of the COST Action as a whole. The momentum created by the new and exciting insights and collaborations that have been generated is continuing, into new activities and funding that are building on the work of the original team and into the future. As McCallin has observed, in the context of nursing engagement in interdisciplinary research:

Interdisciplinary researching is complex and potentially risky; however, it does offer the opportunities for professional growth, development, and research work satisfaction. (McCallin, 2006: 2008)

It has been noted that the formation of effective interdisciplinary teams depends as much on emotional intelligence and positive relationships (including the sharing of humour) as it does on practical organisation and leadership (Giacomini, 2004; McCallin and Bamford, 2007; Nair *et al*, 2008). This state of the art book demonstrates what is possible in this multidisciplinary-transdisciplinary continuum when emotional intelligence, good humour, and positive relationships meet in a critical dynamic with what Pawson has referred to as *'a mutually monitoring, disputatious community of truth seekers'* (Pawson, 2013: 191). Indeed, the Action included not only academics and scientists, but also policy makers, services users, and childbirth activists. Being constructively disputatious in this context allows for an alignment of diverse professional and disciplinary identities and philosophical norms and outlooks with an intention to maximise wellbeing and to take account of multiple perspectives and drivers. This is evident in the book itself, which acts as a demonstration of the concepts of salutogenesis and complexity. Fractally, these attributes were also evident in the Action as it developed and matured. Since the Action has been completed, these relationships and mutual activities have continued to grow and develop, in ways that have been emergent and unexpected. We look forward to the exciting and, as yet, unknown consequences for new, important knowledge, and for optimal maternity care, in the future.

References

Choi BC, Pak AW (2006). Multidisciplinarity, interdisciplinarity and transdisciplinarity in health research, services, education and policy: 1. Definitions, objectives, and evidence of effectiveness. *Clin Invest Med* 29(6): 351-364.

Giacomini M (2004). Interdisciplinarity in health services research: dreams and nightmares, maladies and remedies. *J Health Serv Res Policy* 9(3): 177-183.

Klein JT (2006). Evaluation of interdisciplinary and transdisciplinary research: a literature review. *Am J Prev Med* 35(2 Suppl): S116-123.

McCallin AM (2006). Interdisciplinary researching: exploring the opportunities and risks of working together. *Nurs Health Sci* 8(2): 88-94.

McCallin A, Bamford A (2007). Interdisciplinary teamwork: is the influence of emotional intelligence fully appreciated? *J Nurs Manag* 15(4): 386-391.

Nair KM, Dolovich L, Brazil K, Raina P (2008). It's all about relationships: a qualitative study of health researchers' perspectives of conducting interdisciplinary health research. *MC Health Serv Res.* 23(8): 110.

Pawson R (2013). A mutually monitoring, disputatious community of truth seekers. In: Pawson R: *The Science of Evaluation: A Realist Manifesto*. London: Sage Publications.

Author biographies

Marie-Clare Balaam BA (Hons), MA. Marie-Clare is a research assistant in the Research in Childbirth and Health Unit (ReaCH) at the University of Central Lancashire. Her background is in history and women's studies. Her research interests are migrant women's experiences of maternity care and childbirth in the UK and Europe, social support in maternity care and historical and socio-cultural perspectives on women's health, particularly menopause. Her current research is focused on the experiences of asylum seeking and refugee women and social support for marginalised women.

Cecily Begley RGN, RM, RNT, FFNRCSI, MSc, MA, PhD, FTCD. Cecily is Professor of Nursing and Midwifery at Trinity College Dublin. Her research interests include physiological childbirth and women-centred maternity care. She is a member of national and international research review committees, and has published over 120 peer-reviewed research papers.

Marie Berg RN, RM, MNSci, MPH, PhD. Marie is Professor in Health Care Science specialising in reproductive and perinatal health at the University of Gothenburg (UGOT), Sweden, including working as a clinical midwife at Sahlgrenska University Hospital. Marie is the leader of the childbirth research group at UGOT Institute of Health Care Science. She has led and is leading several research projects with a variety of research designs. Marie has published around 75 scientific papers, several book chapters and a few books. Major research areas: midwifery model of care; labour management; diabetes and pregnancy / childbirth.

Sarah Church PhD (Midwifery), MSc (Research), PGDipEd, PGCertResSup, RGN, RM, SFHEA. Sarah is Associate Professor and Reader in Midwifery at London South Bank University, London. Sarah has contributed journal articles and book chapters on issues within the sociology of reproduction and childbirth. Her PhD focused on gender identity and explored the reproductive identities and experiences of midwives and mothers. Current research areas: lesbian motherhood, perinatal mental health and migration and midwifery, especially migrant midwives.

Jette Aaroe Clausen PhD (Science and Technology Studies). Jette is a Senior Lecturer on the Midwifery program at Metropolitan University College, Copenhagen, Denmark. Her research focuses on the use of technology in childbirth and she is one of the authors of Planned Hospital Birth versus Planned Home Birth in the Cochrane library. She is also engaged in work on Human Rights in Childbirth.

Declan Devane PhD, MSc, PgDip (Stats), BSc, DipHE, RGN, RM, RNT. Declan is Professor of Midwifery at NUI Galway and Director of the Health Research Board – Trials Methodology Research Network (HRB-TMRN). He is an Editor with the Cochrane Pregnancy and Childbirth Group and an Honorary Senior Lecturer at Cochrane UK. Declan has published over 100 papers including numerous Cochrane systematic reviews, predominantly in the field of fetal assessment. He has led a number of clinical trials recruiting from 100 to over 3000 participants and serves on a number of Trial Steering Committees and Data Monitoring Boards.

Soo Downe BA (Hons), RM, MSc, PhD, OBE. Soo is Professor of Midwifery Studies at the University of Central Lancashire, Preston, UK, and she was the Chair of EU COST Action IS0409. She is interested in the utility of complexity theory in understanding dynamic health states. Her specific focus is the normal physiology of childbirth, including the processes which can maximise normal birth, with a focus on the understanding of the nature of positive wellbeing (salutogenesis) as opposed to simply reducing pathology. She is a member of a range of national and international strategic bodies, and she has published more than 90 peer-reviewed papers.

Lucy Frith BA (Hons), MPhil (Cantab), PhD. Lucy is a Reader in Bioethics and Social Science at the University of Liverpool. She has taught healthcare ethics to medical students and healthcare professionals for a number of years. Her research focuses on the social and ethical aspects of healthcare decision-making, policy and regulation, with a particular interest in empirical ethics and socio-legal approaches. She has carried out research on pregnancy and childbirth; reproductive technologies (gamete and embryo donation); research ethics (clinical trials and public involvement and cross-cultural issues in consent); the organisation and funding of healthcare provision; and the use of evidence in practice and policy. She has held visiting fellowships at the Centre for Research in Arts, Social Science and Humanities (CRASSH) at the University of Cambridge and the Centre for Medical Ethics and Law at the University of Hong Kong.

Helga Gottfredsdottir RN, RM, PhD. Helga is an Associate Professor in Midwifery and Head of Midwifery Studies at the Faculty of Nursing, University of Iceland. She is also a Director of research and development regarding pregnancy and antenatal care at the Faculty of Nursing. She has published scientific papers and book chapters at an international and national level.

Olga Gouni. Olga is a Whole-Self Prenatal Psychotherapist/Educator. She is the Founder/Dean of Cosmoanelixis, a service offering prenatal and life sciences online education in Athens. She is the external educator for the Kapodistrian University (EKPA), Athens, the Founder/ President of the Hellenic Union for Prenatal and Perinatal Psychology & Medicine, and Co-Director for Greece & Cyprus for the Whole-Self Discovery & Development Institute, International. Her main interest is connecting the academic world with the community designing and implementing services that promote human evolution and peace.

Mechthild M. Gross RM, RN, BSc, MSc, Dr, PD. Mechthild is the Director of the Midwifery Research and Education Unit at Hannover Medical School. She is the head of an MSc programme for midwives which is part of the European Master of Science in Midwifery. Mechthild has published widely mainly on early labour, women's experiences and high-risk pregnancies during labour.

Barbara Kaiser PhD. Barbara is a Professor at the HES-SO University of Applied Sciences, in the Midwifery Department of the School of Health Sciences, Geneva, Switzerland. Her main perinatal research areas include health behaviours during the post-partum period, complementary and alternative medicine for pregnancy-related health conditions and midwife-led units.

Annette Kuhn PD, Dr. Med. Since 2000 Annette Kuhn has been a consultant in uro-gynaecology at the Inselspittal Bern. She studied medicine in Hannover and at the same time undertook studies in philosophy and history, also in Hannover. Apart from undertaking various advanced training courses, her medical career has been spent in Switzerland where she is active in a number of professional organisations, currently holding the presidency of two important Swiss organisations working in the field of uro-gynaecology. She remains particularly interested in ethical issues concerning cowmen's health and diminishing resources. She is a member of the Cantonal Ethics Commission for Bern.

Bengt Lindstrom MD (Pediatrics), Phd, DrPH, Professor of Salutogenesis, Chair of IUHPE Global Working Group on Salutogenesis, NTNU, Norway. Main area of interest in this COST project: implementation of the saluotogenic framework in childbirth and maternity care.

Ans Luyben, RM, PGDEd, PGDM, PhD. Her background is midwifery and health and social science. Ans is a midwife in the Women's Clinic, Spital STS AG Thun and an independent international consultant in maternal and child health and education. She is an honorary lecturer at the Department of Health Services Research, University of Liverpool, and a visiting research fellow at the School of Health and Social Care, Bournemouth University. Publications can be found in a variety of Dutch, English, French and German professional journals and books, and her research interests involve organisational system design and culture, women's experiences and person-centred care, antenatal care and cross-national comparative studies.

Anne Lyberg, RN, RPN, PPHN, MNSc. Anne is Professor in Nursing Science at the Centre for Women's, Family and Child Health, University College of Southeast Norway. She has published several scientific papers in the area of maternity care with a focus on leadership and management, mental health and migrant health.

Irene Maffi is Professor of Social Anthropology at the Institute of Social Sciences, University of Lausanne. She is the author of *Women, Health and the State in the Middle East. The politics and culture of childbirth in Jordan* and one of the editors of *Accompagner la grossesse et la naissance. Savoirs et pratiques professionnels en Suisse romande.*

Claudia Meier Magistretti DPhil, PhD is director of research at Lucerne University of Applied Arts and Sciences, Department of Social Work. She is a clinical and health psychologist with the main research areas in efficacy measurement, maternity and early child care, diversity in health, prevention and health promotion. She is also a visiting professor in several Universities in Switzerland and Austria.

Karin (CS) Minnie, M Cur, PhD. Karin is the Director of INSINQ Research Focus Area at the Potchefstroom campus of the North-West University in South Africa. She is a Registered Nurse and Midwife Specialist. Her research focus is on knowledge translation to improve the quality of nursing and midwifery care.

Marianne Nieuwenhuijze RM, MPH, PhD. Marianne is head of the Research Centre for Midwifery Science at Zuyd University Maastricht in the Netherlands. She is the leader of a number of projects on childbirth research and has published scientific papers on physiological childbirth, client participation, shared decision-making, health promotion and public health.

Mercedes Perez-Botella, RN, RM, MA, PGCert Ed. Mercedes is a Midwifery Lecturer at the University of Central Lancashire, UK. She is also part of the Research in Childbirth and Health research group at UCLan and has published some work around maternity care and also higher education in the UK.

Mário J. D. S. Santos MSc is a research assistant in Sociology at the University Institute of Lisbon (ISCTE-IUL), Portugal. He has a degree in Nursing, an MSc in Health, Medicine and Society (2012) and is currently a PhD candidate, focusing on the social dynamics of the professional and informal home birth networks in Portugal. His main research interests are: gender, the (de)medicalisation of childbirth, and home birth.

Valerie Smith, PhD, RNT, RM, RGN. Valerie is a part-time Lecturer in Midwifery at the School of Nursing & Midwifery, Trinity College Dublin, and a part-time Research Fellow at the School of Nursing & Midwifery, National University of Ireland, Galway. Valerie's specific clinical and research interests and expertise are in methods for assessment of fetal wellbeing, outcome measures in maternity care, normal childbirth, randomised trials and systematic review methodology. Valerie has published widely on the topic of fetal assessment, and on salutogenically focused outcome measures, sexual health after childbirth, preterm birth and risk in maternity care.

Edwin van Teijlingen, MA, MEd, PhD. Edwin is Professor of Reproductive Health Research at Bournemouth University, UK. He is a medical sociologist and has published over 200 papers, several books and over thirty book chapters. His research includes studies on various aspects of the organisation of maternity care and midwifery. He is also Visiting Professor at two colleges affiliated with universities in Nepal.

Berit Viken, RN, RPHN, anthropologist is Associate Professor and researcher at Centre for Women's, Family and Child Health, Faculty of Health Sciences, University College of Southeast, Norway. She teaches in a master's program in health promotion and in the bachelor program in nursing and is the leader of a further education course in supervision and coaching. Her research interest is migration and health, with a special focus on health services in a multicultural society.

Acknowledgements

First and foremost we would like to thank the European Union for funding our project through COST Action IS0907. This edited collection is one of the key outputs of COST Action IS0907.

Working across Europe and beyond is only possible if people collaborate effectively. We have been very fortunate in our COST Action that so many good people have contributed in face-to-face meetings held in the UK, Malta, Ireland, Finland, Portugal, Belgium, Serbia, the Czech Republic and Greece, as well as in phone calls and on-line. This book is the culmination of many people's thinking, contributions to face-to-face discussion across Europe, telephone conferences, and email exchanges. We thank all those who have helped us in any way and at any time during the four years of COST Action IS0907.

The editors

Index